G000077958

Weakness Became Strength
Copyright © Nov 2020

Unless otherwise indicated, all Scriptures are taken from the Bible in the following translation: Message translation (MSG), King James Version (KJV), New King James Version (NKJV), Amplified Bible (AMP), New Living Translation (NLT), New American Standard Bible (NASB), Good News Bible (GNB) and NIV translations (NIV).

ISBN:

Published by
London, England
Printed in the UK

Layout by
Bishopforte

Table Of Contents

Acknowledgement

There's an African proverb which says, "It takes a village to raise a child." What this means is that it takes many people (not just family) to help with the nurture and growth of an individual and that has been the journey of my life which birthed this book.

A big thanks goes to my wonderful parents, Mr. and Mrs. Yinka Odunubi, who gave me life and sacrificed daily for me to become who I am today. Without both of you, there would be no me. Thank you for your love and support over the years.

Also, I want to say thank you to my wonderful siblings Bayo, Deji, Bose and Muyiwa, knowing you all and seeing you all grow up has been such a joy to behold.

There are countless people who believed in me and helped me over the years. I would like to thank those who helped me birth this book and also played a tremendous role in my spiritual life as a Christian. Pastor Gabriel Onyekwelu, thank you for actively investing in my spiritual growth over the years; your advice, encouragement and wisdom in the last few years have greatly affected the daily choices I make for the kingdom of God. Thank you for your teaching that actively promotes having an intimate relationship with God which has shaped my spiritual growth and set me on the right path. To Mrs Bimpe Onyekwelu your support, encouragement, and advice in birthing this book from start to finish is much appreciated; when I didn't know the next step to take before and during the writing of this book, you always showed up with great wisdom and ideas on how to keep moving forward. Thank you for challenging me to think out of the box. Thanks also to Kemi Adeniji, for the sisterly role you play in my life; you always come to all my speaking engagements, cheering me on and also believing the best in me.

Thank you to my amazing and special friends Bayo, Bisi, Seun, Teju and Toni for all your wonderful encouragement and support over the years.

Thank you to my church family Genesis Chapel, for giving me room to grow in different capacity.

A big thank you to my editorial team Tola Awe and Ayo Oyeniji; writing a book is one part but finding a team that can read your mind, give you great advice and ideas that will lead you in the right direction is another. Thank you being part of my journey.

Finally, to all those who read this book and pass it on to someone whom you believe it will inspire, encourage, motivate, transform and be victorious, THANK YOU!

Dedication

This book is dedicated to the One and Only true God, who held my hand when I was weak emotionally, physically, financially, and spiritually. The One who formed me, created me, called me by name, chose me, appointed me, and predestined me before I was formed in my mother's womb. The One who chose not to give up on me when I had given up on my life. He, who whispered into my ears, "I will make your weakness to become strength" The One who did exceedingly and abundantly above what I could ever think or ask for.

Lord, I am forever grateful for all You did and will do in and through my life. Thank you, Daddy; my heart will forever long for You all the days of my life.

Foreword

"I have known Seun personally for over a decade. I met her at a time in her life when the idea of weight loss was "unthinkable". Back then, I was utterly taken by how tall, dark, striking, confident and majestic she looked, and carried herself, and even more after her weight loss. If you want to read a book that will give you a reason to seek out a healthy lifestyle, then this is the book. I can certainly say she has written the truth – unembellished and unexaggerated, because I witnessed her entire transformation. This is an inspirational read and I hope you are as motivated and delighted reading it as I was witnessing her Journey."

Adebayo Akande, MBBS, SNSH Dip (Nutrition & Herbalism)

....

It would be an understatement to say that this book 'Weakness Became Strength', is nothing short of an honest, inspirational, and heart-warming memoir of Seun's weight loss journey. It is much more than that. Having known Seun for over twelve years and counting, I am proud to say that I was privileged to witness, first-hand, her weight loss journey – the highs and the lows, the pains and the triumphs that make up this candid and well-put-together account of how it all started, and how exactly she overcame issues of low self-esteem, lack of self-control, inferiority complex, identity issues and obesity; issues that we are all too aware, often overwhelm a myriad of people in this world.

Weakness Became Strength has a lot to offer both believers and unbelievers alike, through its stories, sound and godly counsel, tried and tested practical tips, and research-based facts. Are you struggling with obesity, lack of self-control, low self-esteem, identity issues and the like? Then you want to get a copy of this book and learn how to attain victory from someone who has, and till today, is still a living testimony of what she's written in her book.

Bimpe Onyekwelu, Co-Pastor Genesis Chapel (RCCG), Author of "IDENTITY: Discovering Your New Identity in Christ".

I must say it was a bolt out of the blue when I was asked to write this but I daresay, having been an ardent observer of Seun's transition when she was under my tutelage in a previous ministry assignment; it's a great pleasure to do so. Many will pick up tips from this book on how to lose weight or get into better shape physically which, I must say, is a great start to healthy living.

Here, the author guides readers through a journey of discovery which enabled her to find herself, connect with her maker and focus on the understanding that all things could be done by the God who strengthens her.

She chronicles the peaks and troughs of her quest with great intrigue and bare honesty which should encourage anyone going through a similar travail that they can do it too! The essence of this book and the main takeaway is that healthy living is not an event, but a lifestyle choice based on definitive habits (hourly, daily, weekly, monthly etc.); the fact that we've been fearfully and wonderfully made by God does not negate the personal responsibility that we have to cultivate and maintain our physical being.

I'm a firm believer that individuals are the best marketers of their products if they epitomise them and I can testify that Seun has not just adjusted favourably in her quest to live a healthy lifestyle but, as she has over the years, maintained her target status quo and thereby become a great advert for all the measures she took and is proffering for others to follow.

Enjoy the rollercoaster read that will give you the spiritual, emotional, and physical, emotional wherewithal to overcome the obstacles to change and be the best you.

Ade Adewumi, 'Executive Pastor', The Liberty Church, London

Introduction

Many people are looking for different ways to discover who they really are. The average human being will do anything to discover their purpose in life. Therefore, people often go to different conferences to hear and learn from speakers who have walked the path they want to walk. We invest in several self-help books and sign up for mentorship programmes that will uncover our potential and help us discover our true self.

There is something about man on earth that truly makes him want to know where he came from, why he is here on earth, what his purpose is, what his true potential is and if he is walking on the right path. Some people are still confused, and they do not realise why they are here on earth, others have gone to their graves still asking this question, others wake up every day and they long to discover their true selves, while some others don't even know that God has already mapped out a plan for their lives. This process has led many down the path to depression, suicide, hopelessness, just-existing and just-passing through life each day.

Just imagine this, what if something as simple as making up your mind to lose weight, getting out of debt, changing your habits (with the help of God), can be the chosen path that He has assigned for you to discover your true self? What if choosing to make healthy choices will lead you to the path God has chosen for you? What if choosing to renew your mind with the Word of God daily will lead you to that path? Finally, what if choosing to build your relationship with God, learning to hear His voice daily and obeying Him daily is the key to unlocking your journey so that you start knowing your purpose and path? The Bible says in **1 Corinthians 1: 27 – 30, NIV:**

"But God chose the foolish things of the world to shame the wise; God chose the weak things of the world to shame the strong. God chose the lowly things of

this world and the despised things—and the things that are not—to nullify the things that are, so that no one may boast before him. It is because of him that you are in Christ Jesus, who has become for us wisdom from God—that is, our righteousness, holiness and redemption."

Like the examples given above, simple life decisions can be the path that will lead you to purpose because the God that we serve is good at choosing things that don't necessarily make much sense to the human mind. He uses such things to show Himself mighty and strong.

I am glad that I made up my mind about nine years ago to lose weight. At the time, my life was filled with so much hopelessness, depression, anxiety, and worry. I was in debt and I didn't believe in myself or my ability to do anything. The feeling of rejection, insignificance or unworthiness was my constant companion, and my self-image was very poor. I looked at my life and contemplated whether life was worth living – did I really have any purpose on earth? Why am I here? It was during this period of confusion that I found God. I decided to show up in church one morning and I paid attention to the pastor's message and thus a new journey started. I am still on that journey of self-discovery in Christ till today.

Right now, at this very moment, I am a totally different person who has been healed and restored emotionally by God. Through His grace, all the negativity mentioned above is history. Here I am today, giving encouragement to women and anyone who feels they don't deserve much, or feels less valued or wanted. I can honestly say that God will make your weakness become strength. God can and will turn your mess into a message and He will turn your disadvantage into an advantage.

By embarking on this journey with God, I discovered who He created me to be. I discovered I am good enough, that I have a purpose on earth, that there are many great things about me, and I am still discovering these things daily. I am not where I want to be, but I am no longer where I use to be, and I am pressing on.

Let me first encourage you, by letting you know that surrendering your weight loss struggles or changing your lifestyle with the help of God is one of the best decisions you will ever make. God does not start or get involved in something that fails. In the past, you might have failed a few times or given up like I did, but it all worked because God never let me go and He keeps empowering me daily with grace.

The Bible says in **Philippians 1: 6, NIV:**

   "Being confident of this, that He who began a good work in you will carry it on to completion until the day of Christ Jesus".

God began it and authored it, and whatever He authors is always good. In the book of **Genesis 1: 31, NIV,** when God finished the creation, the Bible records:

   "God saw all that he had made, and it was very good."

The Bible calls Him the Good Shepherd; you can see that the nature of God is good. Most importantly though, the good work He begins in us will always start from the inside first and then work its way until it reflects on our outside.

Allow God to lead you one day at a time as He led me; and note that the road He may lead you on may not make sense and may even look like another person's journey. Therefore, it is important that you trust Him completely and at the end you will be transformed from the inside out. He will make your weakness become strength and turn your mess into a message.

Book
One

A Wake-up Call Answered By Faith

"GOD, did You tell me that I can do all things through Christ who strengthens me? Does that include weight loss, settling my debts, believing in myself, being all You created me to be, gaining freedom from childhood trauma, being set free from suicidal thoughts and depression? Lord, You must be joking', I said.

I made these statements in disbelief based on what I thought possible with my natural ability. I had fallen into a pit of despair and my mind could not comprehend a situation where I would be able to emerge from it. I can only imagine what the Lord thought of my utterances! Thank God for His unconditional love, mercy, and grace that I have through Christ Jesus.

One day I woke up feeling fed up. I got out of bed, looked at myself in the mirror and I said "Seun you can't continue like this!" I had a light bulb moment and for the first time in my life, it occurred to me that I could lose weight with help from God and that I could also overcome all the challenges I had been dealing with Yes! I COULD LOSE WEIGHT WITH HELP FROM GOD – not by 'trying' to lose weight. I didn't have any plan or desired goal about the journey, but I knew that I was ready and willing.

I believe God helped me realise this because I was about to begin a journey of self-discovery; I was on the threshold of something that was bigger than me. I didn't have a clue about what to do or even how to go about it. All I remember is that I had made up my mind to lose weight and by God's grace, I was going to find a way to do it.

What I didn't know that day, was that God had plans for me and He was going to take me through a journey that I could never have imagined for myself. The book of **Jeremiah 29: 11, AMP** states:

> *"For I alone know the plans and thoughts that I have for you,' says the Lord, 'plans for peace and well-being and not for disaster, to give you a future and a hope".*

Well, peace and well-being (the state of feeling happy, comfortable, and healthy) were very far from me! Just a few months before this time, I had been in a very dark place going through periods filled with suicidal thoughts, depression, anxiety, worry, insecurity, low self-esteem – you name it, I had it.

I had lost my job after spending six years with an organisation I thought supported me. It was the first time in my life I had been out of work. I remember thinking *"Seun, you are not good enough, that is why they let you go"*, *"Seun, you are overqualified for your job."*

From the moment I was sacked till the moment I handed over all keys and property that had been in my custody to my former employer, many different thoughts went through my mind. In hindsight, I realise that the experience was just a steppingstone towards greater things, and I have not looked back since then.

If I'm honest with myself, my job had become my identity and my image. Consequently, I felt as if things went downhill for me after that day. The fake exterior I had built over the years through my job was slowly dismantled. To say I was shattered would be an understatement. I can now see God worked it all out for my good; He used that bad situation and turned it around for good. He needed to strip me of the identity I had created through my lifestyle (of then) which was all about my façade and very superficial (what kind of job I had, what school I went or where I lived etc) and give me the real one in Christ, which is

3

eternal and can never be taken away from me.

I realised that I had to start looking for another job, this time in a different field. It was hard, lonely, and depressing. I had never been unemployed in my life so pushing through that season was difficult. Life as I knew it became tough and I could barely cope as I felt constantly overwhelmed with fear. Most days, I didn't even feel like getting out of bed, I was dejected as a result of the constant rejections I had received while job hunting. During this time however, I slowly found my way back to GOD.

I remember my pastor, Pastor Gabriel, preaching one Sunday and he talked about having a relationship with God. It felt kind of weird because this was the first time in my Christian life that my ears were opened to knowing and accepting that I needed to have a relationship with God. I believe that I paid attention to Pastor Gabriel that morning because I had been under a lot of pressure and I had become desperate for help. I mean, I needed God to come through for me ASAP! I had heard so much of "You need to have a relationship with God," "You can talk to God about anything," "God is interested in the small and big things in your life," "God will rescue you from any hardship you are currently going through, He is a good father and He alone had an amazing plan for your life even before you were born." I thought, "Okay! Let me give God a try."

At first it felt very strange, I was full of doubt, fear, and uncertainty. I had so many questions! How do you talk to God and have a relationship with Him? Do you just wake up and start talking to God when you can neither see Him nor feel Him? How do you know He hears you and how do you know you can rely on Him? What does His voice sound like? Does He really talk? What is His character like? How will God respond when I call on Him? Can I call on Him at any time? How do I even call on Him? I didn't have any answers to these questions, but I was willing to give an intimate relationship with God a try. At that point I didn't have any other alternative.

Before this time, I would describe myself as someone who was deeply religious. I was in and out of different churches on Sundays even though I claimed I was a born-again Christian. I would go from one church programme or conference to another (I was a church fornicator; it feels strange saying this now but that was my reality at the time). Your story may be like mine. Don't worry there is hope for you in Christ Jesus!

Why would I call myself a church fornicator? Well, what I meant was this, even though I had a church I attended regularly, I was one of those people who would always look for one prophet or pastor that would act as a mediator between me and God. I believed they could tell me what God was saying or would either deliver me from one bad dream or the other. I would also be searching for the next Christian conference or program in town. I used to have nightmares constantly, I knew that something wasn't right. I was frequently on the phone hoping to find the latest deliverance prophet in town or I would move from one deliverance service to another. I remember I once went all the way from London to Birmingham for a three-day deliverance service!

I never knew I could have a personal relationship with God and that I could hear Him all by myself and just by knowing, believing, and applying the truth in His word I would be delivered. I never knew that one of the primary ways God communicates with us is through the Bible – His written word. I never knew that I had authority over demons through Christ Jesus. I never knew my mind needed to be refreshed and renewed with the word of God. I knew that I was born again, went to church every Sunday and attended house fellowship. I even joined the evangelism department but that was it, empty activity because I was lacking that direct connection with God. I had misplaced priorities about the things of God because I didn't know better. My goals every Sunday in church were to look good, check the guys out and just meet friends. This routine continued for years. I never knew that developing an intimate relationship with God and knowing him as a Father would allow me to grow spiritually.

I started taking my walk with God seriously and I would wake up to study the Bible daily. For a long time though, it was as if I was reading a story book and, oh boy, I felt like dropping it! After just one week, I remember telling my pastor that I wanted to give up on reading the Bible. He encouraged me by telling me that the way I was feeling wasn't strange and that I should just keep reading, so I persevered. He also suggested certain books from the New Testament that I should start reading including the book of Ephesians, Galatians, Philippians, and Colossians. I am very grateful for his spiritual guidance.

I went back to reading the Bible, but this time I believed that the Holy Spirit would give me understanding. Before I knew what was happening, the word of God started speaking to me and my situation. I was startled initially because I had never had that experience of the word speaking life to me as it did that day. All thoughts of hopelessness, unworthiness, insignificance, anxiety, and depression started fading away. It did not happen overnight, but I noticed that the more time I spent reading, studying and meditating on the word of God, the more peace and joy I felt even amid overwhelming challenges. It was the first time in my life that I realised that God could speak to me directly, before that, I believed God would speak only through a pastor or prophet.

As each day passed by, I began to learn different ways through which God could and would communicate with me. He spoke to me through His written word in the Bible, through the messages I listened to in church, through my private Bible study, through messages online and through a variety of books.

I don't remember having any specific conversation with God about losing weight. I do, however, remember that one day I got out of bed and made the decision to lose weight. I began my walk of faith; it is a decision I am so happy I made.

When I started that walk, I was weak physically, mentally, spiritually, and financially but I knew I was ready to change. I soon found out that God had been patiently waiting for me to yield myself to the process and to trust Him to lead me out of the situation I was in. It was a new thing He was doing – a new thing that started in my spirit, my soul and then worked its way out through my body.

God came through each day. He never for once left my side and every single time I had an obstacle He always showed up through the Holy Spirit, either by comforting me or giving me the wisdom, I needed each day to overcome.

There were many Bible passages that comforted me especially when I felt like quitting. In fact, I gave up a few times, but God always sent His word to me somehow and it gave me the courage to continue. A particular passage I remembered at the time is in **Isaiah 43:19 – 20, MSG** and it states:

"Be alert, be present. I'm about to do something brand-new. It's bursting out! Don't you see it? There it is! I'm making a road through the desert, rivers in the Badlands. Wild animals will say 'Thank you! The coyotes and the buzzards - Because I provided water in the desert, rivers through the sun-baked earth, Drinking water for the people I chose."

Therefore, I knew each day I needed to be alert and this came about through prayers and studying the Bible each morning. The word of God became the source of my strength because it was all that I knew to rely on.

I had never tried to lose weight before and like I said earlier, I didn't have any clue how to go about it. God led me step by step He gave me the gift of faith to lose weight while in a troubled circumstance. Not many people would embark on a weight loss journey amid what seemed to be several insurmountable challenges. In fact, I think it's realistic to say that it's during periods like this that one either gains or loses considerable weight in an unhealthy manner because of worry and the issues of life. So, you either eat to distract yourself or you are unable to eat because of worry. If I hadn't started building my relationship with God, I don't think I could even have attempted to lose weight but with God all things are possible to those who believe. This journey can never be adequately told without emphasising how God was involved.

So please sit back, grab a cup of tea or coffee, make sure you have a note pad and pen; and just open your heart to God. Get ready to laugh, get your faith stirred up and let me show you through this book how my weakness indeed became strength with the help of the Almighty God. If God could do it for me who was once weak, mentally, emotionally, financially, and physically, then He will do exceeding and abundant things beyond all you could ever ask for.

You might have attempted to lose weight repeatedly in the past and it didn't work, you might be going through some financial challenges right now, you might have some mental health illness struggles; and you might have gone through phases of depression, suicidal thoughts, anxiety and worries. This time around it will be different if you allow the Almighty God to be involved and you also allow Him to lead you. Whenever God starts something, He always finishes it, therefore He is called the Alpha and the Omega, the Beginning and the End of all things. Always remember if He could do it for me, He will surely do the same for you because He is your Father, Helper and Deliverer, and with Him all things are possible to them that believe.

Reminder: *Always be rest assured that God is with you on this journey, guiding you each day.* The Bible says in Philippians 1:6, NIV,

> *"Being confident of this, that he who began a good work in you will carry it on to completion until the day of Christ Jesus."*
>
> *God started it and He will complete it; all you need to do is yield to Him and He will ensure you get to the end of the journey.*

The Root Cause-the Emotional Eater

The journey had started, and I did not know the first step to take. My quiet time with God was filled with so many prayers like "Lord I need your help. I don't know what to do, please show me the way." My prayers were quite simple and plain most times as I had just started taking this walk with God. I didn't know much of the Bible then, so I just said what came from my heart. God in His mercy and loving kindness, through the Holy Spirit led me on the right path.

I had so many internal issues or rather, identity issues. I didn't think much of myself as a person, my default self-image was one filled with lack of self-esteem and self-confidence, powerlessness, unworthiness and insignificance.

While I was growing up which continued to my adult years. my mother constantly compared me with other people. I don't know why she did that. She would say "So and so had a better grade", "So and so is slim, and not fat like you", "So and so has a better job" or "So and so has built a house for her parents". My life looked so perfect on the outside but inside I was lost and broken. I felt like something was wrong with me and that was what I had been told all my life. My mother's words had aided in creating wounds – wounds that festered with lack of self-esteem and confidence. Through her words my wall of self-esteem was broken down, I became a prey to the enemy. I didn't believe that I could amount to much in life, and I felt unworthy and insignificant.

The **Merriam Webster Dictionary** defines the terms *'insignificant'* and *'unworthy'* below.

Definition of Insignificant

* Lacking meaning

- Small in size, quantity, or number
- Not worth considering: Unimportant
- Lacking weight, position, or influence: Contemptible

Definition of Unworthy
- Lacking in excellence or value: Poor or Worthless
- Not meritorious: Underserving, unworthy of attention
- Not deserved: Unmerited, unworthy treatment

The words above describe how I perceived myself over the years until I began to know who I was in Christ Jesus.

Frequently while growing up, I felt neglected and abandoned. At the age of 6, I was sent to boarding school. I remembered staying up all night during those early years, wishing my parents would come looking for me or change their minds about leaving me there. I believe they thought at the time that they made the best decision because they were trying to balance their business commitments as well as raising me. However, this choice cost me a lot in my formative years, but my Heavenly Father is now restoring me.

I often felt neglected, I believed that my parents didn't love me and that was the reason they abandoned me. I might not have felt like that had they shown me any form of physical and emotional affection. It was during my healing process that the Lord helped me realise that it was not their fault because they didn't know any better. He made me realise that it is impossible to give what you don't have.

My parent's way of showing affection and love was buying good clothes, providing meals for me, and sending me to a good school. Any emotional connection was non-existent, and this was one of my foundational problems. It was a constant battle. On the outside I looked all put together but, on the inside, I was broken and crushed. Words like "You are beautiful" or "You are Precious" were very foreign to me, and I never heard my Dad or Mum say them to me. I sought approval from the men I dated, approval that I never got. I remember the first guy who told me he loved me. I had never heard that before in my life and I just went with the flow. The feeling of wanting to be loved with no strings attached (sex and money) was rare from the opposite sex. I constantly fell into the wrong hands of men – men who were broke, jobless and lacked any purpose or vision. As the years went by, my self-esteem and self-confidence diminished every day.

I started dating someone and everything looked good and I believed it would lead to marriage. Our parents were introduced to one another but a few days later he dropped a bombshell – he no longer wanted to marry me. I was crushed. What a life I had lived!

Looking back now, I can see that it was all the work of the devil using my upbringing and the bad choices or decisions I made daily to lead me down a dark path. The Bible says, the thief comes to steal, kill and destroy, but I came that you please insert your name here and say it out loud), might have life and have it in abundance (**John 10: 10**). The enemy used my parents' ignorance to prey upon me and because they were authority figures in my life, I believed whatever they said about me whether it was good or bad.

The choices I made when it came to men were all driven by my desire to be loved, feelings of rejection, low self-esteem, lack of confidence and believing others were better than me.

While I was in secondary school I was picked on and bullied constantly. I schooled in Kaduna, which is in the northern part of Nigeria, for six years. It was my choice to stay far away from home because I wanted a different experience from the one, I had become accustomed to living in the south where I grew up.

I was bullied because I was fat as a child. I knew I was slightly bigger than my peers which didn't bother me that much when I was at home. However, when I got to secondary school it really made me a target for bullying. I was told my belly was big and I was even given a nickname. I remember two boys who would call me repeatedly by the nickname and I didn't have the courage to report them. I knew that even if I had reported them there would never have been a positive outcome, so I kept quiet. My grades suffered a lot. I did not enjoy my six years of studying in the north.

My childhood trauma was one of the things God uncovered and helped me to deal with on my journey to self-discovery. **Proverbs 23: 7, NKJV** says,

"*As a man thinks in his heart, so is he.*"

As I pondered over these negative words daily, I became driven by negative thoughts, never for once happy with my life. I wanted to commit suicide at least twice and this unhappiness was the root cause of my emotional eating.

On this journey, God opened my eyes to see that when parents constantly abuse (physically or emotionally), neglect or compare their children to others and always see the worst in their children, they unconsciously strip them of their self-esteem, worth, confidence or purpose. However, when parents speak life into their children by encouraging them, disciplining, guiding, training them in the way of the Lord and building up their identity in Christ; they are building them for the kingdom of God and those children will have a sense of value and self-worth. They will become all that God wants them to be. So, parents which kingdom are you building? Are you stealing, killing, or destroying your children's lives by what you say to them or are you speaking life to them? Always remember that you will reap what you sow. My relationship with my parents has greatly improved and with the help of God I have forgiven them.

There were many things that I had to work through with God and most times I felt like giving up, I didn't give up because He gave me the courage not to on my journey. Before then, my mind had been a complete wreck. I easily gave up on things and I would always look for an excuse not to do what was important. If I felt stressed, I would eat. If things didn't go my way, I would eat. If I felt overwhelmed with anything, I would eat. If I felt dejected about something, I would eat. If I felt unloved after a breakup, I would eat.

Lest I forget I was also bad at managing money and it fuelled my emotional eating habit. When I got my first credit card, a card from Barclay's bank, I thought 'free money!' I immediately went on a shopping spree buying the latest in fashion, filling my wardrobe with clothes and shoes. They were of course impulse purchases; I wanted validation from people and before I knew it, I started acquiring more credit cards and store cards. At a point I took out a loan of about £2,000 for a boyfriend, he never paid me back. I now realise how silly I was.

I had accumulated quite a few credit cards, store cards and loans over the years as a student. I would often fail to make payments. Consequently, I would be fined, and the interest rate went up once I missed a couple of payments. After a while, I just didn't bother to pay anything towards them. Eventually the credit cards and store cards companies came after me because they wanted their money back. Once again, I had given up like I usually did once a situation became too difficult for me to handle. I ended up being pursued by the bailiff for a debt of almost £10,000! Eventually I was able to pay off this debt.

Back then, I was basically what could be described as an emotional eater and I was also a shopaholic. I was not being led by the Holy Spirit but by the impulse of the flesh. I did whatever I fancied and felt like doing at that moment. **Colossians**

3: 5-8, MSG says,

> "*And that means killing off everything connected with that way of death: sexual promiscuity, impurity, lust, doing whatever you feel like whenever you feel like it, and grabbing whatever attracts your fancy. **That's a life shaped by things and feelings instead of by God.** It's because of this kind of thing that God is about to explode in anger. It wasn't long ago that you were doing all that stuff and not knowing any better. But you know better now, so make sure it's all gone for good: bad temper, irritability, meanness, profanity, dirty talk.*"

My life was being controlled by my flesh (my emotions). I didn't know that there was a thing called living by the spirit, a new and regenerated version of oneself, a new creation in Christ that one can becomes. I was just grabbing whatever I fancied and whatever felt good; my life was being shaped by things and not by God in any way. The Bible says that the way of life is connected to death.

What or who is an Emotional Eater?

According to beateatingdisorder.org.uk, an emotional eater is anyone who turns to food for comfort and escape during times of low mood or stress. When someone overeats emotionally, it is an attempt to feel better, to feel comforted or soothed by eating.

According to MedicineNet, emotional eating is the tendency of its sufferers to respond to stressful, difficult feelings or difficult situations by eating, even when not experiencing physical hunger. Emotional eating or emotional hunger is often a craving for high-calorie or high-carbohydrate foods that have minimal nutritional value. The foods that emotional eaters crave are often referred to as comfort foods like *ice cream, cookies, chocolate, chips, French fries, and pizza. About 40% of people tend to eat more when stressed, while about 40% eat less and 20% experience no change in the amount of food they eat when exposed to stress. Consequently, stress can be associated with both weight gain and weight loss.*

From the descriptions above, I could now see that the major reason or one of the contributing factors to my emotional eating was stress coupled with childhood trauma. Food was a source of comfort and escape which I had always been quick to resort to throughout my life. This time I had been bingeing on food and using it as a coping mechanism because I had lost my job; I was in serious debt and just confused about life in general. I don't think I can remember if there was a time in my life that I never felt stressed or overwhelmed about something. My default setting was already stress mode!

I remember that before I lost my job, from the moment I would wake up at 6:00am till the moment I came back home at 9:00pm, I was always stressed out! To make things worse, the kind of job I was doing at the time was laden with a host of challenges – constantly having to meet monthly and regional targets, staff Personal Development Plan (PDP) was being done, ensuring staff had their monthly feedback meetings, managing staff, dealing with staff shortage etc. After getting home from a long day at work, all I would want was to eat a big bowl of white rice with some red pepper stew with either fried beef or chicken. I would buy the food on my way home from work and top it off with a cup of chilled coke. At times, I would go for a bowl of Chinese fried rice or fried chicken and chips.

What a life! It brings to mind a couple of popular Nigerian sayings, 'I can't come and kill myself' or 'Na me kill Jesus?' Now I can look back and laugh at my ignorance! I thank God for giving me the power to overcome emotional eating. The book of **Romans 12: 2 NLT,** says,

> *"Don't copy the behaviour and customs of this world, but let God transform you into a new person by changing the way you think. Then you will learn to know God's will for you, which is good and pleasing and perfect."*

The word *'behaviour',* according to the *Lexicon* dictionary, is defined as the way in which one acts or conducts oneself, especially towards others.

17

The same dictionary also defines the word _'custom'_ as _a traditional and widely accepted way of behaving or doing something that is specific to a particular society, place, or time._

The last Bible passage I gave was one of the many truths that set me free. It made me realise that I had been conforming to the behaviour and custom of this world and not conforming to the pattern of the word of God to deal with any situation I found myself as a Christian.

When the pressures of life (worry, anxiety, stress, trials, temptation etc) inevitably hit, I would run to food for comfort instead of seeking comfort from God. The world conditions us to look for a quick escape route when life packs a punch or it seems to be overwhelming or stressful. Globally people, including Christians, are struggling with addictions such as emotional eating, pornography, drinking and many other things. They are all looking for a way to relieve their daily stress and the only One that has the answer to every single one of these addictions is Jesus Christ.

According to the word of God, we are to seek comfort in God alone. **2 Corinthians 1: 3-5, NIV** says,

> _"Praise be to the God and Father of our Lord Jesus Christ, the Father of compassion and the God of all comfort, who comforts us in all our troubles, so that we can comfort those in any trouble with the comfort we ourselves receive from God. For just as we share abundantly in the sufferings of Christ, so also our comfort abounds through Christ."_

God is first a Father of compassion, He will not only shower us with comfort when we go to Him, but He will receive us with everlasting love and comfort us in ALL our troubles, just exactly as how good earthly fathers will do for their children when their children run to them in every difficult situation. 'All' means every single one of our troubles and the reason He does this is so that we too can pass on that comfort to others. God is so generous with His comfort and He freely gives it to us. He understands us and He knows that living in this world comes with trials and tribulations which Jesus has already overcome for us. Hallelujah!

I had to learn that whenever I feel overwhelmed or stressed regarding a matter, I should seek God rather than food or shopping or other things, to make me feel good.

The scripture from the book of **Romans 12: 2, NLT** also made me realise that I needed to allow God to change the way I thought about myself and situations that made me feel hopeless. Through His word I could confront issues making me feel stressed and overwhelmed, and I would have a better handle on life and be able to control my eating habits.

My way of thinking was about to undergo a renovation. I was somewhat ready as I had already made up my mind to lose weight and give up some bad habits. I was desperate and I knew I could only overcome these obstacles with the help of God. The word of God began to help me change the way I think from that moment on. At first, I wondered how a habit of more than 30 years would vanish. You are probably thinking the same thing too, it can change and will change with the help of the Holy Spirit. I have learnt that with God all things are possible, and He has what it takes to create new things out of nothing (**Romans 4:17**).

Is Stress Good or Bad?

According to **stress.org.uk**, *stress is primarily a physical response. When stressed, the body thinks it is under attack and switches to 'fight or flight' mode, releasing a complex mix of hormones and chemicals such as adrenaline, cortisol, and norepinephrine to prepare the body for physical action. This causes a number of* *reactions, from blood being diverted to muscles to shutting down unnecessary bodily functions such as digestion.*

There is no universally agreed medical definition of stress. At its most basic, stress is your body's physical response to mental or emotional pressure. Our jobs, relationships, family life or money, world crises, can all add to our levels of stress.

As earlier stated, when you are stressed, your body believes it is under attack and switches to what is known as 'fight or flight' mode. As a result, a mix of hormones and chemicals are released into your body so that you prepare for physical action. Blood might also be diverted to muscles, causing you to lose concentration or become less able to digest food. When the threat passes, your body usually returns to normal, but if you're continually under pressure this might not be the case. When we experience severe stress, it affects our emotions, physical health, and our behaviour.

Stress can be caused by either the external or internal pressures of life which, the devil will sometimes bring to move us out of the will of God. We could even be the ones also stressing ourselves based on where we think we should be or what we ought to have achieved in life. The book of **John 10: 10, TPT** says,

"A thief (which is the devil) has only one thing in mind – he wants to steal, slaughter and destroy. But I have come to give you everything in abundance, more that you expect – life in its fullness until you overflow!"

This scripture enabled me to see that the devil was (is) after my peace, that which is my spiritual well-being and a gift from God! What the devil was doing in order to steal my peace from me, was to send external pressures of life which would bring me stress and trigger me to lose my peace. This would move me out of the will of God and rather than seeking peace in Him, my solace would be in food, shopping etc. Thank God that His word is truth, and it is now my armour. I now know that it is the truth in the word of God that sets me free. God equipped me with His word daily, as I took time out daily to fellowship with Him by praying, studying the word, meditating on His word, having honest and serious conversations with Him, pouring out my emotions to him daily; I was empowered through His word mentally to fight the good fight of faith to overcome emotional eating.

What are Causes of Stress or Examples of Stress?

- The death of a loved one
- Divorce
- Loss of a job
- Increase in financial obligations
- Getting married
- Moving to a new home
- Chronic illness or injury
- Emotional problems (depression, anxiety, anger, grief, guilt, low self-esteem)
- Taking care of an elderly or sick family member
- Traumatic events such as a natural disaster, nationwide outbreaks (COVID 19), pestilence, theft, rape, or violence against you or a loved one.

Looking at the examples above, I could see the reason why I was always stressed. I had been trying to survive a job loss and at the same time I had unresolved emotional childhood trauma. I had a whirlwind of bad emotions ranging from depression to anxiety, worry, low self-esteem, insecurity, guilt, feelings of insignificance/unworthiness, and rejection. I realised on this journey that God had already given me victory in Christ Jesus over each one of these issues spiritually, but I had to be willing to fight the good fight of faith to experience victory over each one of them in the physical by confronting them with the word of God.

Before I move further, let us consider the statistics of people in the UK that are currently going through stress. As Christians, if we don't know the truth of God's word, then we'll experience the same thing. It is only the truth in Christ that is applied that will set us free from experiencing what the world system is experiencing.

The **Mental Health Foundation** study was conducted in 2018. It was an Online poll undertaken by YouGov and had a sample size of 4,619 respondents. This is the largest known study of stress levels in the UK.

In the past year, 74% of people have felt so stressed they have been overwhelmed or unable to cope.

Age Differences
30% of older people reported never feeling overwhelmed or unable to cope in the past year, compared to 70% of young adults.

Behavioural Effects
46% reported that they ate too much or ate unhealthily due to stress. 29% reported that they started drinking or increased their drinking, and 16% reported that they started smoking or increased their smoking.

Psychological Effects
- 51% of adults who felt stressed reported feeling depressed, and 61% reported feeling anxious.
- Of the people who said they had felt stress at some point in their lives, 16% had self-harmed and 32% said they had had suicidal thoughts and feelings.
- 37% of adults who reported feeling stressed reported feeling lonely as a result.

Causes of Stress

- 36% of all adults who reported stress in the previous year cited either their own or a friend/relative's long-term health condition as a factor. This rose to 44% of adults over 55.

- Of those who reported feeling stressed in the past year, 22% cited debt as a stressor.

- For people who reported high levels of stress, 12% said that feeling like they need to respond to messages instantly was a stressor.

- 49% of 18-24-year olds who have experienced high levels of stress, felt that comparing themselves to others was a source of stress, which was higher than in any of the older age groups.

- 36% of women who felt high levels of stress related this to their comfort with their appearance and body image, compared to 23% of men.

- Housing worries are a key source of stress for younger people (32% of 18-24-year olds cited it as a source of stress in the past year). This is less so for older people (22% for 45-54-year olds and just 7% for over 55s).

- Younger people have higher stress related to the pressure to succeed. 60% of 18-24-year olds and 41% of 25-34-year olds cited this, compared to 17% of 45-54s and 6% of over 55s).

Currently we are experiencing a nationwide outbreak of the COVID 19 virus, the impact of stress on people may reach astronomical levels. The number of people's lives that are being destroyed daily by stress is alarming. As Christians, we are privileged as we have the solution to this problem – Christ Jesus.

Stress itself is not necessarily a bad thing; what can be destructive is the way we go about managing it and seeking freedom from it. Even Jesus said it in the book of John 16: 33, AMP:

"I have told you these things so that in me you may have perfect peace. In the world you will have tribulations and distress and suffering, but be courageous

(be confident, be undaunted, be filled with joy) I have overcome the world. (My conquest is accomplished, my victory abiding)."

What a revelation! Christ didn't sugar coat the troubles of the world we live in, He said 'you will' meaning it will happen. We should be courageous and cheer up because He has already overcome the pressures of this life or whatever this life will throw at us at any given time.

The book of **Isaiah 43: 1- 4,** gives us a perfect picture of how God will continuously be with us in each of our trials in life. He has promised us according to His word that He will never leave us nor forsake us. The scripture gave me more insight and understanding about the pressure of life because it will always be there in one way or another. What stood out for me was the word 'when'. The Bible did not say 'if' you go through trials. It says 'when' meaning it will happen at some point, but the good news is that we can be assured that we will not go down with those trials, because God is with us. We should know that it is a phase which we will pass through and with this knowledge and understanding, we can ride over the storms of life. What is important, is that we know what to do when the storms of life happen.

Isaiah 43: 1- 4, GNT says,

"Israel, the Lord who created you says, "Do not be afraid – I will save you. I have called you by name - you are mine. When you pass through deep waters, I will be with you; your troubles will not overwhelm you. When you pass through fire, you will not be burned; the hard trials that come will not hurt you. For I am the Lord your God, the holy God of Israel, who saves you. I will give up Egypt to set you free; I will give up Ethiopia and Seba. I will give up whole nations to save your life, because you are precious to me and because I love you and give you honour. Do not be afraid—I am with you!"

What a revelation to know about the character of God! The truths above were the foundations that the Holy Spirit laid in my soul to enable me to move forward and face my problems. My situation didn't change overnight, it started changing little by little. With the help of God as I began to behold the truth of His word daily, a renewing of the mind was happening on the inside of me and the root of emotional eating that looked like a Goliath was defeated by applying the word of God to my situation.

Reminder: *Be ready to dig deeper and ask yourself honest questions? Am I an emotional eater? Am I a mindless eater? How did I get here? What can I do to move from where I am to where I want to be?*

The root cause of your weight gain needs to be addressed for you to make progress on your journey. The good news is that God is there all the way to help you to uncover the issues and give you victory!

The Way

Now that I had been able to identify one of my problems – being an emotional eater, it was time to deal with it. I had to take it one step at a time. I renewed my mind daily with the word of God as I didn't have a plan other than to turn to Him. **John 14: 6, NLT** states that:

> *"Jesus told him, "I am the way, the truth, and the life. No one can come to the Father except through me."*

This was one of the truths in God's word, one I stumbled upon while having my morning devotion with God. During this period, I had become desperate and I clung to Jesus; through the above scripture He revealed to me, that He will show me 'the way' out of my emotional eating problems. The Lord became my shepherd and I gladly followed him as a sheep, knowing that the shepherd always has the sheep's best interest at heart.

Social media platforms like Instagram weren't as common in those days as they are now. I think Facebook was the only platform I can remember that most people used, and because it was a new platform, I didn't get any resources about losing weight. I felt prompted to go to Google and search for information about losing weight fast and voila! The Cambridge diet came up. I read a bit about it and I scoffed thinking "I can easily do this, so all I just have to do is drink three shakes in a day, drink plenty of water and the weight will fall off." Who does not like a quick fix?

I believed I had found a way to lose weight, but was it really the way God wanted me to go? Well, I thought this way looked good! The only problem I had was that it wasn't cheap, but it occurred to me that I could still give it a try since I believed that God had made a way.

I read the testimonies of different women describing how the Cambridge diet worked for them and how they were able to lose weight. Their testimonies motivated me enough to want to join and see the immediate result. I filled out the online form and within the next 24 hours, a consultant called me to book an appointment.

By this time, I had been able to get a part-time job, so my financial burden had started to ease. I had also started studying the word of God and I began experiencing victory over suicidal thoughts, depression and the negativity that had previously plagued me. Yes, victory, because I gained knowledge about the many plans God has for my life through His word. I learnt that He is a life-giver not a taker! He had already chosen and accepted me before I was born; Jesus had paid the price for my life and now I belonged to God who had well laid plans for me and those plans were (are) for good and not for evil.

These truths were revealed to me as I spent more and more time with God, studying and meditating on his word daily. In the beginning it was difficult to accept all the good news I was hearing because my thoughts had been rooted in negativity for so long, but that began to change through the Holy Spirit who leads and guide into all truth.

As the days went by, my outlook on life began to change and I started to see myself the way God saw (sees) me. It was a hard and painful process, but I can see the benefits that I am reaping today. The book of **Romans 10: 17, NKJV** says,

"So, then faith comes by hearing, and hearing by the word of God."

The word of faith I received through the daily study of God's word was cleansing my heart as I spent time with Him. It didn't happen overnight; it was a process. As I received truths from the study of God's word daily, the more I noticed I was becoming exactly what the word says I am. One day, while reading the book of

Genesis, I realised something. **The book of Genesis 2: 7, AMP** says,

"Then the Lord God formed [that is, created the body of] man from the dust of the ground, and breathed into his nostrils the breath of life; and the man became a living being [an individual complete in body and spirit]."

God created me in His image and likeness and gave me His breath; then I became a living being complete in body and spirit, lacking nothing. The scripture began to paint a picture of the character of God to me, who He was (is) and it also showed me how intentional God was when He was creating me. As we look through some scriptures below, we will see how God has been a life-giver rather than a life-taker.

Psalm 139: 13–16, NLT

*"**You made** all the delicate, inner parts of my body and knit me together in my mother's womb. **Thank you for making me so wonderfully complex! Your workmanship is marvellous**—how well I know it. **You** watched me as I was being formed in utter seclusion, as I was woven together in the dark of the womb. You saw me before I was born. Every day of my life was recorded in your book. Every moment was laid out before a single day had passed."*

Jeremiah 1: 5, NIV

*"Before **I formed you** in the womb, **I knew you**, before you were born, **I set you apart; I appointed you** as a prophet to the nations."*

I want us to pause a bit here, because I know many people will wonder how I was able to overcome depression, suicidal thoughts, feelings of being unworthy and insignificant, low self-esteem, lack of self-confidence etc. It was the word of God that delivered me completely the more I abided in it daily.

John 8: 31, NKJV says,

*"Then Jesus said to those Jews who believed Him, "If **you abide in My word**,*

*you are My disciples indeed. And **you shall know the truth**, and **the truth shall make you free.**"*

As I abided in the word of God day and night, the more I knew the truth of God's word about me and about the character of God.

Definition of Abide

- To remain, continue, stay.
- To have one's dwell, reside.

Abide means to continue, to stay there and to dwell until you see a change in your thinking pattern. God's word enabled me to see that He had an amazing plan already mapped out for me, plans I couldn't map out for myself. They were already laid out for me.

Ephesians 2: 10, NLT says,

"For we are God's masterpiece. He has created us anew in Christ Jesus, so we can do the good things he planned for us long ago."

Through the scripture, I began to see that God had already mapped out an amazing plan for my life; even my parents couldn't have planned what He had for me.

Another truth that was revealed to me through the above scripture was that God had created a masterpiece in me. I certainly didn't believe I looked like one and I didn't feel like one. Maybe it was a case of mistaken identity, but the more I beheld the word of God daily, the more I began to see myself the way He designed and sees me in Christ Jesus.

The definition of a *'masterpiece'* according to the **Collins** dictionary is

- An <u>outstanding</u> work, <u>achievement,</u> or <u>performance.</u>
- The most outstanding piece of work of a creative artist, craftsman, etc.
- The greatest work made or done by a person or group.
- An artist's, writer's, or composer's masterpiece is the best work that they have ever produced.

This is what God calls us and it is how He sees us forever. You are not a masterpiece, because you behave right all the time, you are a masterpiece because that is your new identity in Christ Jesus, when you became born again and nothing can change it or stop God from seeing you that way. Your identity in Christ is fixed, your circumstance in life might change, you can lose your job or your house, but you can never lose your identity in Christ Jesus as a born-again Christian. Remember knowing who you are is not based on feelings, but on knowing the truth in God's word.

When you know who you are, your behaviour will change, so focus on what God calls you and see how your behaviour changes with time. He still sees you and I as His masterpiece and nothing on earth could change it. You are created and designed by the greatest artist in the world. YOU ARE GOD'S MASTERPIECE!

The word of God began to show me that I was already accepted, approved, appointed, loved, precious, God's masterpiece, a holy nation, a royal priesthood, chosen; in Christ Jesus and there is nothing I can do in this world to earn the love of God. I began to see through the scripture that God treasures me and values me, and therefore He sent Christ to die for me. I was worth dying for, what a revelation!

I am now a child of God; I belong to Him and I have right standing with God through Christ Jesus. It was a beautiful revelation, finding out who I was in Christ Jesus. When I considered the definition of a masterpiece and the scripture above, I began to see myself differently and that changed my attitude and behaviour over a period. My thinking was radically transformed, and my life has never been the same.

I soon found out that it was impossible for God to lie. He can't because He does not have that nature, His nature is to love. It is the devil that is a liar. **John 8: 44, NLT** says,

> "*For you are the children of your father the devil, and you love to do the evil things he does. He was a murderer from the beginning. He has always hated the truth because there is no truth in him. When he lies, it is consistent with his character; for he is a liar and the father of lies.*"

I finally knew who was behind the depression, suicidal thoughts, the feeling of being unworthy and insignificant, all the negativity and it was the devil period! I know this is one area where the world will try and convince you that depression and suicidal is a physical battle; some have even called it mental illness. The devil will always give names to things so that he can distract you from knowing who is behind your issues.

The book of **Ephesian 6: 10 – 13, NLT** states,

> "*A final word: Be strong in the Lord and in his mighty power. Put on all of God's armour so that you will be able to stand firm against all strategies of the devil. For* **we are not fighting against flesh-and-blood enemies, but against evil rulers and authorities of the unseen world, against mighty powers in this dark world, and against evil spirits in the heavenly places.** *Therefore,* **put on every piece of God's armour** *so you will be able to resist the enemy in the time of evil. Then after the battle you will be standing firm.*"

The above scripture made me realise that people and our external circumstances are not the issue or the real enemy, there is someone – the devil and his demons, actively working behind the scenes or people, to cause these issues. Knowing this truth through the scripture above set me free.

Do I still feel attacked or have negative feelings or emotions every now and again? Yes, I do, but the difference now is that I know who I am and whose I am. When the enemy comes with his attacks through people, circumstances, feelings and emotions, I know I need to use the word of God as a weapon of warfare to take those thoughts, feelings and emotions captive into the obedience of Christ.

I meditated daily on the word of God and all the negative feelings began to leave until I came to a place where my mind already had a blueprint of the scripture. It became automatic for me to quote scripture and say it loud each day.

What is Depression?

According to **Mental Health UK**, Depression is a common mental health problem that causes people to experience low mood, loss of interest or pleasure, feelings of guilt or low self-worth, disturbed sleep or appetite, low energy, and poor concentration.

Symptoms:

Depression symptoms may vary among people but generally encompass a feeling of sadness or hopelessness. These can include:

- Tiredness and loss of energy
- Sadness that doesn't go away
- Loss of self-confidence and self-esteem
- Difficulty concentrating
- Not being able to enjoy things that are usually pleasurable or interesting
- Feeling anxious all the time
- Avoiding other people, sometimes even your close friends
- Feelings of helplessness and hopelessness

- Sleeping problems – difficulties in getting off to sleep or waking up much earlier than usual
- Extraordinarily strong feelings of guilt or worthlessness
- Finding it hard to function at work/college/school
- Loss of appetite
- Loss of sex drive and/or sexual problems
- Physical aches and pains
- Thinking about suicide and death
- Self-Harm

Causes:

Depression is a complex condition, and its causes are not fully understood. However, various contributing factors can lead to depression. These can include biological factors (for example, genetics or experience of physical illness or injury) and psychological or social factors (experiences dating back to childhood, unemployment, bereavement, or life-changing events such as pregnancy). Having a long-standing or life-threatening illness, such as heart disease, back pain or cancer, has been associated with an increased risk of depression.

Source - https://www.mentalhealth.org.uk/a-to-z/d/depression

From the definition, symptoms and causes of depression given above, does depression exist? Yes, it does! Can it be cured through the word of God? Yes, it can.

The Bible says in **Proverbs 4: 23, AMPC:**
> *"**Keep and guard your heart** with all vigilance and above all that you guard, for out of it flow the springs of life."*

Proverbs 4: 23, GNT says,

*"Be careful **how you think**; your life is shaped by your*

I had to start paying attention to things that were happening in my life and things I allowed into my heart. What I allowed into my heart, invariably shaped what I thought and what I thought consequently shaped my life. The gateway to your heart is what you see and hear daily, and that is what affects your outlook on life and circumstances. For example, if you consistently expose yourself to bad news regularly, you will not know when you begin to walk in fear, which will lead to worry and anxiety, then lead to depression and before you know it, you find yourself on the slippery road to suicide.

I soon learnt that each time I faced a difficulty or life issues like everyone else, I had a choice to worry and allow anxiety into my life and if I am not careful, it would lead me to depression; or I could go to God in prayer, play worship songs, listen to messages and ask the Holy Spirit to help me. One thing did work – allowing the word of God to take root in my heart daily. It brought about peace of mind, and I became less worried and anxious. Even till today, when worry or anxiety come knocking on the door of my heart, I know what to do.

Depression, suicide, and negative thoughts come with a feeling of helplessness and hopelessness about life. We know, however, that as Christians we now have hope and help in God based on the death, burial, and resurrection of Christ, which is the good news or the gospel. It is not a physical battle; it is first a spiritual battle. From the scriptures given earlier, it is obvious that daily, one must put on the armour of God for one to resist the devil.

I realised that I couldn't be passive in life as I had been in the past. I had to learn to fight the good fight of faith by meditating on the word of God daily and confessing it until my mind was renewed. I had to learn to discipline my mind, my mind was very uncontrollable and always seemed to be busy and wandering!

You don't just wake up one day feeling depressed or suicidal! I have found out that there are always underlying issues that trigger these thoughts, moods, or ways of thinking. In my case, I had unresolved childhood issues and I'd also lost a good job; these were triggers for me. It is common that things like this (depression) start off with a little bit of worry and anxiety, feelings of being unloved/ unappreciated, having no self-worth and feelings of loneliness. Once you sit down and meditate on these thoughts for long, you find yourself depressed – a depression that comes with heaviness of the soul and may take you down that slippery path leading to suicide. No one wakes up one day and just decides to commit suicide! The seed must have been sown and when watered over a long period of time, it bears fruit which is death.

I often hear people say, 'my depression', 'my bipolar disorder', 'my anxiety', 'my childhood trauma' and each time I hear these things, I am quick to correct them and share with them biblical truths. I let them know that those sicknesses and infirmities are no longer theirs as they are born again Christians saved by Christ Jesus. The Bible says it in the book of **Isaiah 53: 4- 5, NIV:**

> *"Surely, he took up our pain and bore our suffering, yet we considered him punished by God, stricken by him, and afflicted. But he was pierced for our transgressions he was crushed for our iniquities; the punishment that brought us peace was on him, and by his wounds we are healed."*

The scripture above shows us that Jesus Christ, our Lord and Saviour, did the following for us

- Took our pain
- Bore our suffering
- Was crushed for our iniquities and
- By His wounds we are healed

This is good news indeed! Christ has already taken all your pain, sufferings, and iniquities; there is no doubt about that. When Jesus Christ was crucified on the cross, He took with Him all your sufferings, all the pains you will ever encounter in this world, they are no longer your own! By faith in the finished work of Christ, you are now free to live a life with no depression, anxiety, worry, bipolar disorder or any other ailment whatsoever. It is high time we believe ourselves dead to these things irrespective of the emotions or feelings connected to them and begin to live the abundant life Christ came to give us. It is no longer 'my depression', 'my childhood trauma', 'my bipolar', 'my anxiety' or whatever name you choose to call it. Just remember Christ took all these things with Him to the cross and by His wounds on the cross, you have been healed. You are now a new creation in Christ Jesus and old things have passed away because God said so. Declare it with your mouth daily, become a student of the word of God and see yourself walking in this truth daily.

Although the Bible doesn't use the word 'depression' except in a few translations and verses, it's often referenced by other similar words, such as downcast, broken-hearted, troubled, miserable, despairing, and mourning, among others. Throughout the Word, there are several stories about godly, influential men and women of faith, who struggled and battled through dark times of hopelessness and depression such as David, Job, Jeremiah, and David. You can read through the highlights of their experiences below.

David was troubled and battled deep despair. In many of the Psalms, he writes of his anguish, loneliness, fear of the enemy, his heart-cry over sin, and the guilt he struggled with because of it. We also see his huge grief in the loss of his sons in **2 Samuel 12: 15-23 and 18: 33.** In other places, David's honesty with his own weaknesses gives hope to us who struggle today:

"Why are you downcast, O my soul? Why so disturbed within me? Put your hope in God for I will yet praise him, my Saviour and my God." **Psalm 42: 11, NIV**

Elijah was discouraged, weary and afraid. After great spiritual victories over the prophets of Baal, this mighty man of God feared and ran for his life, far away from the threats of Jezebel; and there in the desert, he sat down and prayed, defeated and worn out:

"I have had enough LORD," he said. "Take my life; I am no better than my ancestors." **1 Kings 19: 4, NIV**

Job suffered through great loss, devastation, and physical illness. This righteous man of God lost literally everything. So great was his suffering and tragedy, that even his own wife said,

"Are you still holding on to your integrity? Curse God and die!" **Job 2: 9, NIV**

Although Job maintained his faithfulness to God throughout his life, he still struggled deeply through the trenches of pain:

"Why did I not perish at birth, and die as I came from the womb?"
Job 3: 11, NIV

Even Jesus was deeply anguished over what lay before Him. He knew what was to come. He knew that God had called Him to a journey of great suffering, He knew what must happen for us to live free. Our Saviour and Lord was willing to pay the price on our behalf, but it wasn't an easy road. Isaiah prophesied that Christ would be

"A man of sorrows and acquainted with grief." **Isaiah 53: 3, NKJV**

We can be assured, no matter what we face, Jesus understands our weaknesses and suffering, our greatest times of temptation and despair, because He too travelled that road, yet without sin. In the garden, through the night, Jesus prayed, all alone, calling out to His Father, asking Him for another way:

"And He said to them, 'my soul is deeply grieved to the point of death; remain here and keep watch.' And He went a little beyond them and fell to the ground

and began to pray that if it were possible, the hour might pass Him by. And He was saying, 'Abba! Father! All things are possible for You; remove this cup from me; yet not what I will, but what You will.'" **Mark 14: 34-36, NASB**

The Bible says that so great was his anguish, that he sweat "drops of blood." As seem in **Luke 22: 44, NIV:**

During their seasons of hopelessness, discouragement, despair, anxiety and frustration, God was there in the good days and in the dark days too. He didn't condemn them for their questions and pain. He didn't tell them to just tough it out. He reached down to their deepest pit of suffering and lifted them out. He cared. He showed them compassion. He offered mercy. He brought hope. He instilled purpose. He gave victory.

God had provided a way out for me spiritually in the revelations above, He also provided a way out in the physical for my weight loss.

Off I went two days later, and I arrived at Mrs Kimberly's, the Cambridge Diet Consultant and she was gracious enough to answer all my questions. She reassured me that I was on the right track. I was given two weeks' supply of supplements which cost me about £50 to £100 a week and I was told to come and weigh in every week.

With what I believed to be the right product in my hand and believing this was the way God had provided, I was ready to begin but deep down inside I also felt that I should have waited or looked for another way.

Proverb 14: 12, NLT says,

"There is a path before each person that seems right, but it ends in death."

There was something inside of me telling me not to go ahead, but I thought I should at least give it a try. Over the years I have come to learn that God will often prompt us with that feeling deep inside regarding an issue and it is in our best interests that we listen because He knows what is best for us.

I started the plan and gave up after one week! I was constantly tired, and I was always thinking of junk food. I was very miserable. I remember the day I quit very well and that was the best decision I made. At that point, I came to the end of relying on myself.

I went to God again, "Lord, I thought You said You are the Way? Why didn't this way of eating work?" What a question I asked God! How would this way of eating work when I was constantly tired and thinking about all the junk food, I said I wouldn't eat anymore?

Of course, this way of eating didn't work for me because that wasn't the way He wanted me to overcome emotional eating. God may lead us on entirely different routes on our weight loss journeys. This way of eating might have worked for someone else, but it was not for me. Thank God I learnt my lesson quickly and humbled myself before Him to ask for the way forward.

I spent some time praying and asking God for help again. I never gave up on the journey. I was quite surprised at myself that I could be steadfast on this journey because I had a history of quitting whenever things got hard for me to bear.

The Bible says in the book of **James 1: 5 AMP:**

> *"If any of you lacks wisdom [to guide him through a decision or circumstance], he is to ask of [our benevolent] God, who gives to everyone generously and without rebuke or blame, and it will be given to him."*

I asked for divine wisdom because I really didn't know what to do and who I could go to. I really need to emphasise how vulnerable I was during this period of my weight loss journey because that was also when I saw the saving grace of God so much. He lavished me with His grace and strength each day even though my circumstances weren't great, He held my hand, day in and day out. God is good!

A few days later, I was led by the Holy Spirit to call my friend Bayo and I told her about my plan to lose weight, and that I needed her help. She was surprised and laughed at me so hard because she thought I wasn't serious. We had lived together for a few years and she knew better than anyone about my eating habits. I was the chief consumer of junk food! Each time we went out, I was always the hungry one buying Gregg's sausage rolls on the go, buying £1.99 chicken and chips, or clutching a pack of biscuits in my hand.

Bayo, on the other hand, always cooked her meals and would usually keep fruit in her bag as a healthy snack. She was a medical doctor, and she was very health conscious. I remember living with her and each morning she would do some stretching and Pilates exercises (I was always laughing at her and telling her she was wasting her time). I had noticed that she never ate the way I did; my eating habits were bad. I felt her lifestyle was weird. What I didn't know back then was that I was the one living in ignorance. Now that I had called her, I had to humble myself and do whatever she told me to.

She was the answer to my prayers. She led me to the NHS choices website to get more knowledge on eating healthy and portion control. That was how I got to know about the 'Eat well plate'. It was a lifesaver for me because I had never practiced portion control. I never knew we were to portion control our food! I know that sounds funny, right. I was really living in ignorance!

I had crossed my first hurdle, then I moved on to the different types of vegetables to eat. At that time, the only vegetable I had been eating was spinach and it was because it was an ingredient, we used to cook vegetable soup. Even though I knew what carrots and cabbage were, I had never grown up eating them. Vegetables like broccoli, cauliflowers, kale, swiss chard, leeks, and purple cabbage were new to me. I had never eaten or seen them before in the supermarket. I'm proud to say now I know how to eat (I will talk about this more in a different chapter) and what my plate should look like; that was another hurdle crossed.

Even though I had crossed this hurdle of finding a new way of eating, it was still new to me but now I had an idea of what to do before even seeing the result. The next day I made it to the supermarket with my shopping list and on my arrival, I was too embarrassed to ask for help. I thought people would make fun of me if I told them that I couldn't identify certain vegetables – I didn't know what they looked like. Once again, I called my friend Bayo and she assured me it was okay to ask for help. I eventually swallowed my embarrassment and asked for help.

When I got to the vegetable aisle and I was given some broccoli, I called Bayo and told her, "I can't eat broccoli. The head looks like spirogyra!" She laughed at me, but she was also patient and kind, and God knew I needed that kind of grace on my journey. She encouraged me to buy it and go home to either stir fry it or steam it. I was reluctant but I needed help and I had also made up my mind to lose weight. I began to embrace being open to change and knowing that my old ways of living had to die in order to experience the new way of living.

I bought some other vegetables like sweet corn and peas and went home. I had sweetcorn, peas, carbs, and protein as well as the Eat well plate guide! After five days, I got bored! Meanwhile, I hadn't touched the broccoli in my fridge.

Why am I writing this? Simply because I want you to see my struggles in the beginning; I didn't allow any one of them to stop me from doing what I had made up my mind to do. I struggled with knowing what to do or how to go about it, but

41

I asked for help. Don't be embarrassed to ask for help on your weight loss journey. It will save you a lifetime of error and it will end your struggles.

After five days of looking at the broccoli in the fridge and searching the internet for ways to cook it and make it tasty, I worked up the courage to cook it. Since that first bite I took, I have never looked back!

This journey has taught me to confront my fears. Imagine if I never overcame the fear of eating something new, I would have totally missed out on experiencing a new way of eating and at the same time missed out on the nutritional benefits of broccoli.

Now that I had found the way on my second attempt with the God sent help of Bayo, now the real work had begun.

Reminder: *There is always a way out no matter what circumstances you find yourself in this life with Jesus. Jesus is the way, when you lean and follow Him, you can never be strained. There is a way out of whatever circumstances you might be facing be it depression, contemplating suicide, being overweight or health problems; once you fix your eye on Jesus, He will show up.*

Habits

I have learnt that people are born with potential, but it takes challenges and commitment to develop positive habits that reveal the potential within them.

In chapter 2, I discussed how I was able to identify some bad habits of mine – emotional eating and shopping. There isn't a better way to describe some of my old habits – they were bad. I was an emotional/impulsive eater and shopper. I was also unreliable, I would give several reasons for not doing what I knew I ought to do or if I felt something might be too difficult for me, I would just give up. That was one of many habits I had to work through with God, and it was painful, because I had never disciplined my flesh before, but I knew something good was going to come out of it, if I stayed the course. The book of **Hebrews 12: 11, AMP** says,

> *"For the time **being no discipline brings joy, but seems sad and painful**; yet to those **who have been trained by it, afterwards it yields the peaceful fruit of righteousness** [right standing with God and a lifestyle and attitude that seeks conformity to God's will and purpose]."*

Disciplining my flesh brought out so much pain and sadness, it was hard, and I often felt like giving up. I had to learn how to discipline my appetite, my emotions, my mind, and my body. The thought of not being able to buy and eat what I felt like eating was painful to my flesh but looking back now it was a blessing. The good news was that the Holy Spirit helped me through it all. It wasn't easy, but it was worth it.

I discovered that I needed to replace my bad habits with good habits, and I was willing to do this little by little. Thank God for His grace and kindness towards me because He walked me through it daily. It was hard, but I refused to quit in the process. I often say that if you know the root of your problem, you have already solved half of it.

Habits can be described as routine behaviour done unconsciously on a regular basis. They are recurrent and are acquired through frequent repetition.

Let me give you an example, whenever I had a stress trigger what I would generally crave was a bottle of chilled coke to make me feel better or I would go shopping. I had subconsciously done this through the years, so it became a habit. I didn't really need to think about it before grabbing a bottle of coke or going shopping. It had become automatic for me.

'Seun is stressed' = A bottle of coke to calm down

'Seun is feeling down' = Go shopping for clothes or shoes to make you feel better.

The **Collins** dictionary defines the word *'habit'* as:

- A tendency or disposition to act in a particular way.
- An established custom, usual practice.
- Psychology – a learned behavioural response that has become associated with a particular situation, especially one frequently repeated.
- Mental disposition or attitude.
- A practice or substance to which a person is addicted or the state of being dependent on something e.g. drug or food.

From the above definition, we can say the following:

- It is a behaviour
- It is learned
- It is repeated frequently
- It is a mental disposition
- It is a particular way of living

Now that we know what a habit is, let us see how it can be formed.

44

In his book, *The Power of Habit*, author Charles Duhigg explains that every habit starts with a psychological pattern called a "habit loop". The habit loop is a neurological loop that governs habits. The habit loop consists of three elements: a cue, a routine, and a reward.

I had to understand each one of these elements to be able to form new habits. The loop consists of a cue/trigger, routine and then reward. The cue/trigger tells our brain to go into automatic mode. This can be something such as always reaching for junk food, drugs, or cigarettes, when we are under stress. It's a behaviour that neuroscientists have identified as being made in the basal ganglia part of the brain. My trigger was stress or the feeling of being overwhelmed by a task, the reaction – reaching out for junk food then became the routine behaviour without really making any effort to think about it. My reward came from feeling a bit better after eating the junk food, but the feeling didn't last, and the cycle continued.

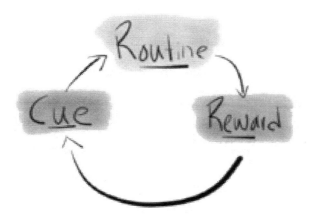

The Holy Spirit became my guide (I was very helpless, in terms of how to change my habits) and my go to person. The word of God in the book of **1 John 2: 27, AMP** says,

*As for you, **the anointing [the special gift, the preparation]** which you received from Him remains [permanently] in you, and you have no need for anyone to teach*

*you. But just as **His anointing teaches you [giving you insight through the presence of the Holy Spirit] about all things,** and is true and is not a lie, and just as His anointing has taught you, you must remain in Him [being rooted in Him, knit to Him]."*

The scripture above spoke to me and I began to ask God how I needed to personalise this new information about forming new habits. Another scripture that ministered to me was **John 16: 13, NLT** which says,

*"When the **Spirit of truth** comes, he will **guide you into all truth**. He will not speak on his own but will tell you what he has heard. He will tell you about the future."*

Who is a Guide?

The **Collins** dictionary defines the word *'guide'* as

- A person who shows the way to others.
- A person who advises others, especially in matters of behaviour or belief, or an adviser, mentor, counsellor
- Show or indicate the way to (someone).
- Direct or influence the behaviour or development of

You can see that the Holy Spirit was Who I needed; I had never tried to lose weight before, and all this was very new to me. It was a new path and a new journey, so I had to rely on Him all the way.

One thing God did for me during this journey was to show me (through the scriptures) that the way I was thinking was standing in the way of my progress. The first thing that needed to be addressed were my words.

Like I said before, I had started taking my relationship with God more seriously and His words were beginning to minister to me. The Holy Spirit is our teacher according to the scriptures and He will guide us into all truth if we will take our place each day by having quiet time with God and studying the scriptures.

One morning, I remember reading the Bible story of the man by the well. The story touched my heart, and I knew that God was ministering to me, that I needed to give up my 'I can't' – excuses. I knew what He was saying deep down inside me, I needed to start renewing my mind in alignment to His words for me to gain victory on this journey. **In John 5: 1-10, NLT** the Bible says,

> *"Afterward Jesus returned to Jerusalem for one of the Jewish holy days. Inside the city, near the Sheep Gate, was the pool of Bethesda, with five covered porches. Crowds of sick people – blind, lame, or paralyzed – lay on the porches.* **One of the men lying there had been sick for thirty-eight years.** *When Jesus saw him and knew he had been ill for a long time, he asked him, "Would you like to get well?"* **"I can't, sir,"** *the sick man said, for I have no one to put me into the pool when the water bubbles up. Someone else always gets there ahead of me." Jesus told him, "Stand up, pick up your mat, and walk!" Instantly, the man was healed! He rolled up his sleeping mat and began walking! But this miracle happened on the Sabbath, so the Jewish leaders objected. They said to the man who was cured, you can't work on the Sabbath! The law doesn't allow you to carry that sleeping mat!"*

didn't have a problem with *'Do you want to get well?'* because I had already made up my mind to get well by losing weight. Where I had a problem was the mind-set of *'I can't'* because I was relying on my strength to lose weight not knowing that I needed to rely on God's strength instead. What an eye opener! I remembered God's word in **Philippians 4: 13, NLT:**

> *"For I can do everything through Christ, who gives me strength."*

My *'I can't'* changed into *'I can'* progressively as I meditated on the word of God. would say it to myself several times a day *'I can! I can! I can do all things through Christ who strengthens me!'* I needed to get those words into my subconscious mind daily until it became autopilot. It wasn't easy at first, but I never gave up on it. The Holy Spirit was showing me a path of thinking that was new to me. **Proverbs 23: 7, NKJV** says,

"For as a man thinks in his heart so is he."

I was becoming a new person with the words I was saying to myself daily. *If you want to replace a bad habit with a new habit, don't focus on stopping the bad habit, focus on replacing the bad habit with a new or good habit;* or rather walk in the spirit and you will not fulfil the desires of the flesh (**Galatians 5: 16**).

One of the various bad habits I had to replace immediately was my Coca-Cola addiction. I had to replace it with water. Drinking Coca-Cola was everything for me. Once I woke up each morning, I would gladly drink a bottle of coke. Without even thinking about it, my body was calling for it. I went cold turkey – I stopped drinking it. I had been a Coca-Cola addict or maybe I should say a sugar addict! I used to drink two to three 500ml bottles of coke daily (that's about 14 to 21 bottles weekly and 10 to 12 bottles of Lucozade orange drink on the side too). There was a buy one, get one free standing offer from the Boots store next to my place of work. I was a regular shopper! What about the cups of hot chocolate I would also grab on the go from Starbucks regularly?

Looking at the drinks I've mentioned above already, if I were to calculate the amount of sugar, I was consuming daily without knowing, we'd be looking at the equivalent of about 55 teaspoons of sugar. Imagine consuming 55 teaspoon of sugar a day without realising it, you can see just how bad of a sugar addict I was.

I can't remember drinking water that much in my life. My mum had been a Coca-Cola drinks distributor while I was growing up, and coke was readily available for us at any given time. That was where my stronghold of coke started (if you have a stronghold of any food or drink, I advise you to dig deeper to find the reason why you are addicted to it. For some people, it is trauma from childhood, that is one of many ways you can begin to walk yourself out of any food addiction (with the help of God).

It was a stronghold for me because I lived by it and survived on it daily. Drinking water was strange to me, but after my encounter with the word of God that morning (the morning His word revealed that I should replace old habits with new), I gave up drinking coke and God truly gave me the grace to start drinking water and desiring more of it. I no longer have a craving for coke or any type of fizzy drink. I am far from those days where all I craved morning, noon and night was coke. The scriptures say He truly gives grace to the humble **(1 Peter 5: 5-6)**. I had already humbled myself and I could see His grace working on my habits.

God showed me that the way to replace a bad habit with a good habit was to focus on developing the good habits and the bad habits would inevitably disappear. Now that I knew the Holy Spirit was my guide and He would always lead me into all truth and that my old habits could be replaced by focusing on building new habits, I began to see that I could conquer and have victory over emotional eating by building new habits and learning new ways of living life.

I've said it repeatedly, it was difficult in the beginning because the idea of forming new habits was new to me; but I was willing to do all I could on my part and allow God to do His part.

I soon learnt that the first 2 - 4 four weeks of building a new habit are usually the hardest. After this period, it gets better and that really helped my confidence on the journey.

According to **Psycho Cybernetics** by Maxwell Maltz, a plastic surgeon who noticed his patients seemed to take a minimum of 21 days to get used to their new face, so the start of forming a new habit takes a minimum of 21 days. However, it takes between 66 days to 365 days to form new habits depending on how the habits have been ingrained into your subconscious mind.

Philippa Lally is a health psychology researcher at University College London. In a study published in the **European Journal of Social Psychology,** Lally and her research team decided to figure out just how long it actually takes to form a habit. The study examined the habits of 96 people over a 12-week period. Each person chose one new habit for the 12 weeks and reported each day on whether they did the behaviour and how automatic the behaviour felt. Some people chose simple habits like "drinking a bottle of water with lunch." Others chose more difficult tasks like "running for 15 minutes before dinner." At the end of the 12 weeks, the researchers analysed the data to determine how long it took each person to go from starting a new behaviour to automatically doing it.

The Answer?

On average, it takes more than two months before a new behaviour becomes automatic — 66 days to be exact; and how long it takes a new habit to form can vary widely depending on the behaviour, the person, and the circumstances. In Lally's study, it took anywhere from 18 days to 254 days for people to form a new habit. In other words, if you want to set your expectations appropriately, the truth is that it will probably take you anywhere from two months to eight months to build a new behaviour into your life — not 21 days.

Interestingly, the researchers also found that "missing one opportunity to perform the behaviour did not materially affect the habit formation process." In other words, it doesn't matter if you mess up every now and then. Building better habits is not an all-or-nothing process.

Now that I knew I needed to replace good habits with bad habits the real work started. There were so many things that I had to replace:

- Eating junk food – Eating healthy or Real food
- Drinking Sugary drinks – Drinking water
- Drinking hot chocolate – Drinking green tea and fruit tea

- Biscuits, cake, pastries – Fruits, nuts etc
- No exercise – Exercising 30 to 40 minutes a day
- Endless TV time – Reading inspirational books or spending time with God
- Panicking after a stressful Day – Going to God for comfort or getting some rest
- Allowing my emotions to control me – Learning to manage my emotions or speaking to God
- Uncontrolled/Unregulated eating (or what I call mindless eating) – Portion Control
- Impulse shopping – Making a list of what I needed and waiting to pay cash for each item
- Lack of Self-discipline/self-control – Exercising self-control/self-discipline

Look at that exhausting list, you can imagine the burden I put on myself. Thank God with the help of the Holy Spirit, I was able to face each problem as I yielded to His prompting on what to do daily. He guided me by giving suggestions and advice, through books or inner witnessing. I must be truthful, although I yielded, there were times I just wanted to throw in the towel, cry, scream and have a pity party. Fortunately, I didn't, and it was not by my ability, but through the help of the Holy Spirit because I had made up my mind to embark on this weight loss journey.

One habit that was a stumbling block for me was exercising. In 2008, I paid £24 a month for a two-year contract for a gym membership and I only went twice! Let's do the maths. That was £576 for a two-year membership. To be honest, I just wanted to go to the gym for fun and be like the Joneses! After that ordeal, I made up my mind that I wasn't going to the gym at all, and God truly made a way out of no way. It really amazed me, how God opened doors of opportunities when I made up my mind to do things His way.

Once again, I went to my friend Bayo and asked for help. I wanted to know what exercises to do and what not to do. I was also counting on the fact she had already gotten used to me asking her some silly and random questions; and even so she was gracious enough to answer me. Bayo opened my eyes to the world of exercise videos and directed me to a website which was later shut down called exercise TV. It was all new and extremely exciting to me. I went online to the Amazon site to order my first exercise video by Jillian Michaels called **30-day Shredder.** A few days later it was delivered, and I started.

I remember money was a bit tight for me at the time and I just couldn't afford to buy a new set of workout clothes. I looked into my wardrobe and found some old t-shirts I had. I also found an old pair of cycling shorts that I casually wore at home whenever I wanted to do some cleaning. For footwear, I came across an old pair of Nike trainers I had, and I was ready to go.

By now, there weren't really any obstacles to stop me from getting into shape. The lack of money, lack of outfits and lack of motivation couldn't stop me. God had used all the hindrances I had faced to teach me that He would always create a way out of no way if I asked Him and relied on Him for guidance. I had given up drinking coke by this time and I had embraced drinking water. My eating habits were getting better and better each day. My emotions were under control and my mind and moods were stable. The next thing I had to do was to face this exercise challenge for the next 30 days and see what would happen to my body.

On day one, I gave up five to seven minutes into the exercise video. I would start again and give up again. I was out of breath, panting heavily and my heart was pounding; but I knew the reason was because I hadn't exercised in a long time. I called Bayo again after I was able to rest and I told her what had happened. She laughed so hard then said, "Seun if the exercise is hard and painful, you can rest in between your workout, but you must always finish whatever you started!"

Really? Finish what I started?

I realised early on that the reason I would always run to her was for a pity party! I didn't have anyone who would really understand my plight like she did because she had also gone through the same experience of losing weight. Bayo wasn't having it and her words killed my excuses, they were life to me, and I still live by them. I say them to myself all the time, I say them to the ladies I am coaching all the time *"You are allowed to rest during your workout but you must always finish what you started."*

I have come across lots of people trying to lose weight who would start but never finish, giving one excuse or the other. Losing weight can feel hard (it's simply because you haven't done it before, but the feeling will leave you when you don't pay too much attention to it and you begin to reap the benefits) if you have so many emotional issues to deal with regarding food. Yes, it can feel hard in the beginning because you are leaving an old way of living to embrace a new one; and when certain challenges come along, you will feel like throwing in the towel and not bothering at all. It is so easy to start anything in life, but it takes guts to be a finisher. You do not develop perseverance, discipline, patience, self-control, or consistency just by starting something in life. You only develop these character traits during the process and that is often where many quit, give up or feel overwhelmed.

I learnt not to be a quitter when things got hard (remember I use to be a quitter). Some days would be good, and some days would not go as planned but I discovered that the only way to get to the finishing line was to enjoy the process and ask God for wisdom and guidance. Thus, I became relentless on my journey by encouraging myself and I also got lots of support from my friend Bayo.

One story that really encouraged me was the story of a man called John Stephen Akhwari, born in 1938 in Mbulu, Tanganyika. He is a Tanzanian athlete and former marathon runner. He represented Tanzania in the Men's Marathon, at the 1968 Summer Olympics in Mexico City. During the marathon, Akhwari experienced severe muscle cramps due to the high altitude of the city. He had never trained at such an altitude before. There was jockeying for position between some runners at the 19-kilometre point of the 42 km race and Akhwari was hit. He fell, seriously wounded his knee, and dislocated that joint. He also hit his shoulder hard against the pavement (can you imagine the excruciating pain?). Nevertheless, he continued running and was the last among the 57 competitors who managed to complete the race out of 75 competitors who had started the race. Mamo Wolde of Ethiopia won the race finishing in 2:20:26 Akhwari finished more than an hour later in 3:25:27, when the majority of spectators had left the stadium and the sun had set. When news came that there was one more runner, Akhwari, was about to finish a television crew was sent out from the medal ceremony. As he crossed the finish line a cheer came from the small crowd that had gathered. During an interview later, Akhwari was asked why he continued running, he said, "My country did not send me 9,000 miles to start the race; they sent me 9,000 miles to finish the race."

What an extraordinary example of a man of integrity, he didn't stop despite the injury he encountered on the way, he kept on going. I can just imagine what was playing on his mind as he kept going despite the pain that he had to endure. I'm sure he must have kept telling himself each step he took "I am going to finish what I started, I didn't come this far to quit. My injury will not stop me, my pain will not stop me. Even if there is no one in the stadium, I will keep going. Tanzania is relying on me to finish. I might not have been the first, but I will finish what started." I'm sure these words or something similar were playing on his mind as he continued running. The Bible says as a man thinks in his heart, so he become **(Proverbs 23: 7).**

In 1983, Akhwari was awarded a National Hero Medal of Honour. He lent his name to the John Stephen Akhwari Athletic Foundation, an organisation which supports Tanzanian athletes training for the Olympic Games. He was invited to the 2000 Olympics in Sydney, Australia. He later appeared in Beijing as a goodwill ambassador in preparation for the 2008 Games. He was a torchbearer in Dar es Salaam, Tanzania on April 13, 2008, for the Olympic torch relay through his country.

All this happened because he refused to quit even when he faced difficulty! Could his name have been written in history as an extraordinary man if he had given up? Absolutely not! His life story is a lesson for us all to see that something good always happens when we refuse to give up on any task that God has given us to do, be it weight loss or something entirely different.

Bayo's words to me *"Seun you must always finish what you started"* became my motto for life because I know "I can do all things through Christ who strengthens me" (**Philippians 4: 13, NKJV**).

Reminder: *A change of one habit can transform you and push you in the right direction for life. You can change with the help of God if you don't give up.*

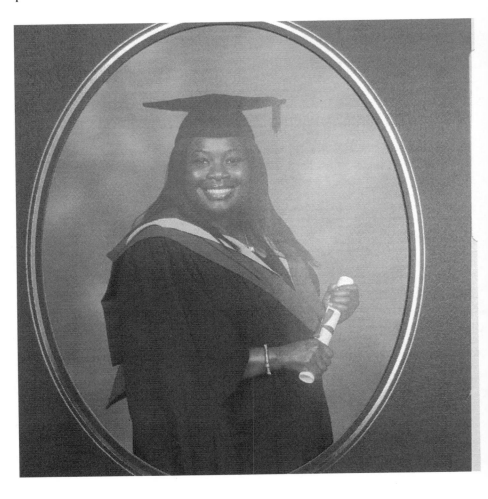

2009 Graduation

The Mind–the Powerhouse

What is the mind?

The **Macmillan** dictionary defines the word *'mind'* below:

- The part of you that thinks, knows, remembers, and feels things.
- Your attention or thoughts.
- Your usual way of thinking.
- Your intelligence and ability to understand things.

If there is one area, I would recommend for anyone to pay more attention to, it is your mind. The battles of life take place in the mind every second, every minute and every hour. In fact, they take place daily from the moment you wake up (including your weight loss battle). Our mind is where victory or loss take place and you can determine the outcome by what you allow into it daily. What you see and hear consistently affect your mind. Your mind is a treasure house, and you have to guard it daily.

Dr Caroline Leaf is a communication pathologist and cognitive neuroscientist. In her book called *'Switch on your Brain'* she talks about our mind being the most powerful thing in the universe after God and I totally agree with her.

Rather than investing in clothes, house, or cars, I have learnt to invest in my mind by feeding it with the right words and aligning it with the word of God. Once you start investing in your mind by filtering what you allow into it at any given time, be it through your eyes and ears and you align it to the word of God, your life can never remain the same again.

Proverbs 4: 20, NIV says,

> *"My son pay attention to what I say, turn your ear to my words. Do not let*

them out of your sight, keep them within your heart; for they are life to those who find them and health to one's whole body. Above all else, guard your heart (mind), for everything you do flows from it."

Are you thinking of losing weight, getting out of debt, becoming emotionally stable, growing spiritually or maybe just accomplishing something good in your life? Then be ready to pay attention to what is going on in your mind. What you hear and what you see are two of the many gates into your mind.

Always remember as you think, so you become. If you think you can't lose weight, you won't but if you think you can lose weight, you will lose the weight and keep it off. You might start off doubting yourself a lot, like I did. You might feel helpless at times, you might even ask yourself "What did I get myself into?" The journey initially might be filled with a lot of fear and hopelessness but don't allow it into your mind. Doubt will tell you all sorts of stories like "You are joking, you can't lose this weight", "Just be content with your current weight", "You have big bones in your family", "You can't give up this and that food", "You're an addict and you will be an addict for life", "You can't come out of debt, you don't have self-control", "People like you can't achieve things like this, there is no point trying" etc. All those thoughts and emotions are part of the journey and as you take each step forward and focus your attention on the word of God, these words will begin to fade away and you will begin to see that you can do whatever God tells you to do through His strength.

In 2005, the **National Science Foundation** published an article about human thoughts per day. According to their research, the average person has about 2,000 to 60,000 thoughts per day. Out of those, 80% are negative and 20% are positive while 95% are the same repetitive thoughts as the day before.

Just imagine that, naturally if you don't reprogram your way of thinking, it is impossible to lose weight and even attempt to do anything great in this world. If you are going to lose weight and keep that weight off, it starts and ends with the mind. That is where lasting transformation starts and takes place. Once you have made up your mind and you stand by your decision, you are going to be transformed forever. Remember that there will be a lot of resistance and challenges on the way, but with the help of God you will overcome that if you choose not to give up.

It took me a while on my journey before I began to embrace this revelation because it was strange to me. The Holy Spirit led me into all truth by helping me understand through the scriptures why I needed to pay more attention to it. My mind was weak, it was a junk house. I believed everything that was spoken into my life. I didn't know I had the power within me to guard my heart and not allow whatever people said to get to me. I didn't know that the only truth I really needed to believe about myself was the word of God. The more I spent time with the word of God, the more my mind was being renewed. I started reading books on the mind, and I became very radical about learning what the mind was all about and how it functioned. I searched the scriptures to find out what the Bible said about the human mind and how God had designed it to function. I came across scriptures like the following.

Romans 12: 2, AMP

> *"And do not be conformed to this world [any longer with its superficial values and customs] but be transformed and progressively changed [as you mature spiritually] by the renewing of your mind [focusing on godly values and ethical attitudes], so that you may prove [for yourselves] what the will of God is, that which is good and acceptable and perfect [in His plan and purpose for you]."*

Philippians 4: 8, NIV

> *"Finally, brothers, whatever is true, whatever is noble, whatever is right,*

whatever is pure, whatever is lovely, whatever is admirable – if anything is excellent or praiseworthy – think about such things."

Colossians 3: 2, NIV

"Set your mind on things above, not on things on the earth."

1 Corinthians 2: 16, NIV

'For "who has known the mind of the LORD that he may instruct Him?" But we have the mind of Christ.'

2 Timothy 1: 7, NKJV

"For God has not given us a spirit of fear, but of power and of love and of a sound mind."

These scriptures about the mind were what God ministered to me. I meditated and affirmed them during and even after my weight loss journey. I still go back to them every now and again because I know the word of God is new each time you behold it. The more I did this, the more I was able to stand the pressures of life, stress and feeling overwhelmed. These scriptures strengthened me and fortified my mind.

Through these scriptures the Holy Spirit showed me that

It is my responsibility to always guard my mind.

It is also my responsibility to renew my mind daily with the word of God.

I have the power to cast down wrong thoughts through Christ Jesus.

I must choose to focus my mind on things that are noble, pure and lovely – that is the word of God.

I must set my mind each day on the word of God and by doing that I enjoy life and peace.

I must be spiritually minded.

- I have the mind of Christ.
- I have a sound mind.

My mind had been a junk house constantly filled with negative thoughts. Before my day would even start, I would have already projected that I would have a bad day. I didn't know I had the power to choose my thoughts until I read a book by Joyce Meyer called *"Battlefield of the Mind"* (if you are currently dealing with depression or worry or any mind-related issues, please read the book). In the book, she talked about how all life battles are won in the mind and how the only weapon we need to use to fight this battle is the word of God. With God's guidance I slowly began to win the battle of the mind.

Lessons Learnt

You Have the Mind of Christ: This was one of the first revelations I had. One thing I have found out through the word of God is that we have been blessed with every spiritual blessing. According to the book of **Ephesians 1: 3, NIV**

> *"Praise be to the God and Father of our Lord Jesus Christ, who has blessed us in the heavenly realms with every spiritual blessing in Christ."*

For me to experience it in the physical I had to know that I had it first in the spiritual. How did I know this, I happened to be reading the book of **Corinthians 2: 12-16, NIV** which says,

> *"What we have received is not the spirit of the world, but the Spirit who is from God, so that we may understand what God has freely given us. This is what we speak, not in words taught us by human wisdom but in words taught by the Spirit, explaining spiritual realities with Spirit-taught words. The person without the Spirit does not accept the things that come from the Spirit of God but considers them foolishness and cannot understand them because they are discerned only through the Spirit. The person with the Spirit makes judgments about all things, but such a person is not subject to merely human*

*judgments, for, who has known the mind of the Lord to instruct him? **But we have the mind of Christ.***"

The scripture above showed me how I came to have the mind of Christ. The mind of Christ does not automatically manifest in us once we become born again. When we become born again (by declaring Jesus is the Lord and Saviour of our life) our body and soul (mind, emotions and will) are still the same, what becomes born again is our spirit. Our spirit is immediately made brand new like God's! That is why the Bible says if any man be in Christ Jesus, he is a new creation, old things have passed away and all things have become new **(2 Corinthians 5: 17, NKJV).**

Our mind can only progressively become new when we begin to constantly renew it with the word of God daily.
The Bible says in the book of **Romans 12: 2, TPT,**

"Stop imitating the ideals and opinions of the culture around you but be inwardly transformed by the Holy Spirit through a total reformation of how you think. This will empower you to discern God's will as you live a beautiful life, satisfying and perfect in his eyes."

For us to experience all the things Christ has freely given, we need to be transformed by renewing our minds. Trust me, it doesn't happen overnight! It is a process which a lot of us are not patient enough to go through. Before we became born again, our minds were filled with the ways of thinking of the world and we were doing things that were against the way of God. However, once we become born again, the Holy Spirit begins to lead us into all truth. As we begin to study the word of God daily, a renovation begins to happen in our conscious and subconscious mind. This process might take months depending on how much time you give to the word of God, and the renewing of the mind is a lifetime process.

In my case, I was very desperate, so I ensured that I spent a lot of time reading, studying, and meditating on the word until I came across a scripture that mentioned having the mind of Christ **(1 Corinthians 2: 16)** and that became my starting point.

Having the mind of Christ wasn't an automatic thing for me but reading and understanding the scripture was where the process of renewing my mind had begun. It was the scripture that also showed me that it was impossible for Christ to be depressed or even have suicidal thoughts, so if Christ never experienced it on earth then I shouldn't allow it or rather, I had to resist feeling negative emotions.

The mind of Christ is not passive, it is disciplined and self-controlled. The mind of Christ is not full of worry or anxiety, it is clear and focused. I had to keep reminding myself each time when my thoughts were all over the place 'Seun you have the mind of Christ so keep it focused.' I would say this affirmation to myself every day. Sometimes I got frustrated and I felt like giving up, but the more I kept saying it the more it was registering in my subconscious mind, till it inevitably became a part of me. Even now at times, I have to remind myself whenever I feel my mind is being attacked or it is wandering, to say it loudly 'Seun you have the mind of Christ.' I know I have it and I will keep fighting the good fight of faith to have all the things that Christ died for me to have in this life.

Set Your Mind: I've said it a few times, my mind was like a Rollercoaster, it was hard concentrating on anything for too long. My mind was not disciplined at all and I knew for me to have victory, this was an area I had to work on. I had made it a mission in life. I didn't know I could set my mind on the right things. I didn't even know I had the power within me to do that. I had to rely on the Holy Spirit to lead me and guide me on this journey of mine as I was clueless.

The Holy Spirit would always lead me to the truth of God's word if only I was willing to spend more time studying it. After realising that I had the mind of Christ, I also needed to know what to set my mind on daily. Knowing the word of God is one step, doing the word of God is another step. This was where the 'doing' part began because it is in the doing that you are blessed, and you have victory. Each day, I had to learn to set my mind on the outcome I wanted for each day.

The **Cambridge** dictionary defines the word **'set'** as 'to put something in a particular place or position.' Therefore, I had to learn to fix my mind or thoughts on the word of God. The Bible says in **Colossians 3: 1-4, NIV,**

> *"Since, then, you have been raised with Christ, **set your hearts on things above**, where Christ is, seated at the right hand of God. **Set your minds on things above**, not on earthly things. For you died, and your life is now hidden with Christ in God. When Christ, who is your life, appears, then you also will appear with him in glory."*

What I learnt from this scripture, was that my mind needed to be set on things from God (things above) such as joy, peace, love, self-control, and abundance among other things. This meant that I shouldn't let the distractions of this world get to me and I needed to start seeing things from God's perspective. Learning to set my mind wasn't an easy task I must say! It took months before I started seeing the results. Each day I would wake up, look to the word of God, meditate on it, and confess it again and again. I didn't realise it, but my mind was being disciplined each day. One day I woke up and I found out that the suicidal thoughts, depression, and negative emotions that had plagued me for so long were all gone!

When I started to see results during this process (setting my mind), I implemented it into my weight loss plan. For example, each morning I would wake up and set my mind by telling myself in advance that "Seun you will only eat this certain food you take to work and nothing else." I knew I couldn't control what would happen at my place of work, but I could control myself by planning my thoughts in advance in case people offered me what I didn't plan to eat on that day. I would set my mind each day before I went out anywhere. Even before going out for any party too, I would do the same thing. I would tell myself for example "You can only eat small chops today." I would also ensure that I had eaten something before I headed out. Whenever I was invited to a restaurant, I would search the menu online first and decide ahead on what I wanted to eat. This really helped me. I noticed that the more I conditioned myself this way, the more I was enabled to say no to different kinds of junk food.

Setting your mind on your weight loss journey might not be easy, but I am a testimony that it can be done. Always remember, we are moving from one level of glory to glory, the Bible says the path of the righteous shines brighter and brighter each day (**Proverbs 4: 18**). It might not happen in a day or even for several months but don't give up. When you see yourself falling, ask the Holy Spirit to help you. The truth is that if you don't give up, the devil will give in because you are fighting from a place of victory and we know that victory is always ours in Christ Jesus.

Take All Thoughts Captive: You can choose your thoughts? Really? What a revelation to me. I remembered reading about it in a Joyce Meyer book, **Battlefield of the Mind.** I thought "Really, I didn't know that." I thought all thoughts that came into my head were mine until I learnt that the devil could inject thoughts into your mind. He did it to Jesus. In **Matthew 4: 1, NLT** the Bible tells us,

> *"Then Jesus was led by the Spirit into the wilderness to be tempted there by the devil. For forty days and forty nights he fasted and became very hungry. During that time, the devil came and said to him, 'If you are the Son of God, tell these stones to become loaves of bread.' But Jesus told him, 'No! The Scriptures say, 'People do not live by bread alone, but by every word that*

comes from the mouth of God."

Yes, Jesus experienced it himself because the Bible says, "the devil came and said to Him." The devil didn't appear to Him in the physical, he spoke into His ears and look at how Jesus defeated him, Jesus spoke back to him to counter the words that he spoke because Jesus already knew the word of God. Imagine if Jesus didn't know that word of God, He would have believed that lie and it would become His reality.

Once I realised this truth, I began to pay attention to my thoughts. I also found out that the more I knew the word of God, the easier it became to recognise the negative thoughts the devil was injecting, I could take them captive and replace them with the word of God.

For a long time, I had believed that I could not amount to much in life, it came with a feeling of not wanting to do much or even trying anything. However, the more I knew the word of God, the more I found out that those thoughts and feelings were not from Him and that God already had a good plan for me whether I felt it or not. One thing God taught me on this journey was never to be ed by my feelings or emotions, but rather by His word.

I began to pay attention to what was going on in my head each second, each minute, each hour, and each day. Even till now, I still do it. I check my thoughts and I always process them through the word of God. For example, if I suddenly have a thought regarding a situation that I have committed to God for a turn around and I find myself thinking that God will not come through, I will take that thought captive by declaring that with God all things are possible, or I might declare "My God will supply all my needs according to His riches in Christ Jesus." I do at times fail at this, but I continue because I know that I am retraining an old mind to think in a new way. That doesn't come easily!

I also had to remind myself that I am no longer where I use to be and that I am moving from one place of glory to another each day. Am I there yet? No! Have I recovered more ground in my mind? Yes! Am I pressing on each day? Yes! I have forgotten those things and left them behind, and I'm reaching for the things in front of me.

What I have explained above is the process of renewing the mind daily. **Romans 12:2, NIV** says,

> *"Do not conform to the pattern of this world but be transformed by the renewing of your mind. Then you will be able to test and approve what God's will is—his good, pleasing and perfect will."*

Renewing the mind is a process, it doesn't happen overnight, and the length of time may be dependent on what areas you have problems in. My problems were emotional eating and overspending. I had to work through so many layers of hurt, forgiveness, frustration, anger, stress, worry and anxiety in my soul each day.

The more time I spent immersed in the word of God, the more my mind was being programmed to start thinking the way I believed God wanted me to think when faced with challenges, and then my new way of thinking began to affect my actions. I am still a work in progress. I am not where I want to be, but I am no longer where I use to be. It is possible to renew your mind with the word of God. It is possible to replace negative thoughts with Godly thoughts. It is possible to move from being carnally minded to being spiritually minded. However, you have a role to play first and the Holy Spirit will guide you into all truth as He leads you to become a new creation.

God wants us to experience the freedom from all addictions that the blood of Jesus Christ bought for us. It is already ours in Christ Jesus, but we need to activate it by faith first, then begin to renew our minds with the help of the Holy Spirit and before long we'll be thinking, talking and acting as God wants us to and we will become unstoppable.

Reminder: *You can choose your thoughts, not all thoughts are yours and the only way you can know if you are thinking the right way is when your thoughts are aligned with the word of God. Changing the way, you think does not happen overnight, it will happen little by little, so don't give up. You can do all things through Christ who strengthens you!*

Self-control

"Like a city whose walls are broken through is a person who lacks self-control." (**Proverbs 25:28, NIV**)

The journey for me was becoming clearer and clearer each day. I felt at this point on my journey that I could handle anything that came my way, through Christ Jesus. The Holy Spirit was always there to guide me. Each day I would declare loudly, "Thank you God for what you are doing." I had begun to have a handle on how to portion control my food and when to exercise, whether I felt like it or not. At some point, I even tried running! Oh yes, I did but I hated it and after two months I gave up. I don't even know why I endured it for that long!

I soon learnt that I needed to try new things with an open mind to see whether they were suitable for me or not. Even at that, I still consulted the Holy Spirit each time. Would I ever try running again? I might because I have learnt to keep my mind open with God. I tried Zumba too. I liked the thought of moving my waist (I was beginning to see that I had one) and twisting my body but I had to stop after the one nearby closed.

I tried different exercises until I found the one that worked for me and that is why I am 'Team Home Workout' because it killed my excuses of "Oh, I don't have a gym membership" or "It is cold I can't go out for a run."

God knew I needed another revelation on this journey that would set me free. One thing I have realised is that the word of God has a way of locating us even amid our trials. A lot of us worry if we will ever hear the voice of God or know the ways of God but He is always communicating with us. There's a need for us to connect with God and recognise when He's communicating. One sure way of knowing this is through His word. The book of **John 10: 27, NKJV** says,

"My sheep hear My voice, and I know them, and they follow Me."
His words will never ever fail, and this is certain if you spend time with him reading and living through His word.

I had started taking my relationship with God seriously, and the desire to fellowship with Him each day before I started my day, was growing stronger and stronger. I came across a wonderful scripture in **Galatians 5: 22- 24, NIV** which says,

> *"But the fruit of the Spirit is love, joy, peace, forbearance, kindness, goodness, faithfulness, gentleness and self-control. Against such things there is no law. Those who belong to Christ Jesus have crucified the flesh with its passions and desires."*

Hold on, did you just say I have self-control Lord? Really?
You are probably amused by some of my utterances whenever I have a revelation from God. I had been fed lies all my life while growing up. I had believed the things people told me about myself! I found that reading and understanding the word of God, realising that He was using that same word to communicate and reveal to me what I have in Him through Christ was truly amazing. When God who created you in His image and likeness tells you that you have something good in you, you had better take it as THE TRUTH and the ONLY TRUTH, even when everything around you contradict that. If God says you have it, there's no argument or debate about it.

I became inspired to study more about self-control. First, I went online to check the dictionary for the meaning of self-control.

On this journey (weight loss), I never even tried to use will power. I didn't even know what willpower was. I feel God made it that way so that I could be completely reliant on Him. It has been the best decision I ever made. Weight loss is a personal journey and God has a personalised and bespoke plan for you to lead you out of any pit you might find yourself in. The book of **2 Peter 2: 9 NIV** says,

> *"If this is so, then the Lord knows how to rescue the godly from trials and to hold the unrighteous for punishment on the day of judgment."*

Only God knows how to rescue the godly from any trials or any problem one might be going through. This was the reason I kept going back and forth to Him all the time.

What is Self-Control?

The **Collins** Dictionary describes '*self-control*' as the ability to exercise restraint or control over one feelings, emotions or reactions or the ability to control oneself, one's emotions and desires, especially in difficult situations.

Other meanings include self-discipline, self-restraint, control, self-mastery, and moderation.

I could hardly believe what I had just discovered. I had been told another truth that would set me free. The Bible says in **John 8: 31-32, NLT,**

> *"Jesus said to the people who believed in him, "You are truly my disciples if you remain faithful to my teachings. And you will know the truth, and the truth will set you free."*

Therefore, I had to remain faithful to His teachings or word. I began to see the benefit of fellowshipping with the Lord because the Holy Spirit was opening my eyes to the truth of the word of God!

Another thing I learnt along the way was that the devil hates us knowing the truth. He loves to keep us in bondage, and he will do anything to ensure we never get into the word of God because he knows if we ever know the truth, his power over us is over.

Hosea 4: 6, NIV says,

"My people are destroyed from lack of knowledge. 'Because you have rejected knowledge, I also reject you as my priests; because you have ignored the law of your God, I also will ignore your children."

Indeed, we are destroyed by the lies of the devil when we don't know that truth of God's words. The Bible says in **John 10: 10, NIV,**

"The thief comes only to steal and kill and destroy; I have come that they may have life and have it to the full."

The devil's work is to steal, kill and destroy our life each day we wake up, and we have the choice to either choose his way or the way of the Lord.

Lord, so I have self-control? I had a weapon to fight with on this journey! I searched for more scriptures regarding self-control and I found the following passage in **Proverbs 25: 28, NIV**

"Like a city whose walls are broken through is a person who lacks self-control."

With each revelation that came to me, I always had this "Oh Lord" moment! I was spoilt for choice like a kid in a candy store. It began to make sense to me as I meditated upon these two passages above. I discovered the following.

The reason I had an emotional eating problem was because my walls had been broken into, the wall of my soul (emotions, will and feelings)! We are a spirit (through Christ Jesus), we have a soul, and we live in a body. The part of us that is the soul, consists of our will, emotions, reasoning, and feelings. That is the part that God wants to work on, and it needs to be renewed with the word of God.

While I had been studying the Bible, my mind was being renewed. It often felt difficult but at the same time, it was effortless because I was not relying on myself alone, I was relying on the Holy Spirit, to teach me and guide me on my journey.

The Bible says a person without self-control is like a city without a wall. Just imagine a city without a wall right now! A city without walls represents a place where anything and anyone is free to roam, to bring in, to leave, to take, to damage, and to destroy anything they choose.

At the start of my weight loss journey, I often felt out of control. The walls of my mind, appetite and emotions were all down. I couldn't walk by a chicken and chip shop and not go in and buy something. If I walked past KFC, I had to buy something. If I saw a cake leftover in the fridge at work, I had to eat it! I had a big weakness for rice. I had to eat a big portion of rice with a bottle of coke EVERY DAY! My motto was you see it, smell it and you eat it.

This is the reason why many of us are slaves to food and we keep eating junk food. I am telling my story to set others free and to let them know they can choose to have freedom in Christ Jesus and indeed be free. My life was a wreck and I made good or bad food choices; there was no distinction. My guard was down! I had discovered the reason why I had a problem; I needed the help of the Lord to help me rebuild these walls. I knew I couldn't rebuild them by myself. This journey helped me expose my vulnerability to the Lord. If you know me well, I am not a person that shows her vulnerability, but this journey brought it all out.

John 15: 5, NLT says,
> *"Yes, I am the vine; you are the branches. Those who remain in me, and I in them, will produce much fruit. For apart from me you can do nothing."*

Apart from HIM, I (can) do nothing – including losing weight! So, I relied on the

Lord to guide me each day.

The second thing I discovered was that I already had self-control within me, it was not something outside of me. It was part of my identity in Christ Jesus, it was who I was, it was given to me freely in Christ Jesus and all I needed to do was to exercise it daily. When I became born again, my spirit became like God's. The old 'Adamic' nature was killed off and a new nature was automatically given to me. My spirit was brand new. Therefore, the Bible says, if any man be in Christ Jesus, he is a new creation, old things have passed away, now OLD THINGS HAVE BECOME NEW (**2 Corinthians 5: 17**). 'He is', meaning ALREADY, the Bible didn't say 'he is going to' be one.

My spirit was brand new, which meant every attribute of God I had in my spirit, the real me. It might not have looked like that in the natural (my physical body) but spiritually I had His nature, character (Fruit of the Spirit) in me. **Colossians 2: 9-10, NLT** says,

> *"For in Christ lives all the fullness of God in a human body. So, you also are complete through your union with Christ, who is the head over every ruler and authority."*

From the above scripture, it means that through Christ, I am complete in Him – lacking nothing. Self-control was therefore in me and not outside of my reach, it is who I am. I often hear Christians say, "I don't have self-control or discipline" and that is a lie from the devil. They often feel that self-control is not within their reach and that one day they may randomly encounter it, but they keep waiting in vain. They have believed a lie and they are living according to that lie. It's because of this that they find it hard to lose weight or exercise self-control in other areas of their life when they need to.

If you are born again then you have the spirit of the Lord living on the inside of you. If Christ Jesus is your master and saviour, if you are a child of God and you belong to the kingdom of God, **YOU HAVE SELF CONTROL** and that is the truth of the word of God. It is part of your redemption right, Jesus paid for it with His blood and it is free to you. You don't need to cry or beg God for it. You already have it in you and all you need to do is to activate it by faith and exercise it daily. It is a daily thing and the more you use it, the more you get stronger and stronger.

Self-control is one of nine fruit of the spirit, and it is given to us when we become born again. **Galatians 5: 22-23, NIV** says,

> *"But the fruit of the Spirit is love, joy, peace, forbearance, kindness, goodness, faithfulness, gentleness and self-control."*

I don't know why self-control comes last on that list but that doesn't really matter now.

How do we have fruit? Every fruit starts with a seed. A fruit does not just appear overnight. Every fruit starts with a seed, when it is sown on good soil and nurtured (in the right climate and watered) it becomes fruit. The Holy Spirit said to me "Seun you have self-control, but it is still a seed. You need to nurture it daily and the more you do that, the more it will grow."

I went to work on it, and I began to meditate on that passage (**Galatians 5: 22-23**) day and night. I was experiencing the instruction given in **Joshua 1: 8, NLT:**

> *"Study this Book of Instruction continually. Meditate on it day and night so you will be sure to obey everything written in it. Only then will you prosper and succeed in all you do. This is my command—be strong and courageous! Do not be afraid or discouraged. For the LORD, your God is with you wherever you go."*

I woke up every day looking at the scripture, I would say it while I was in the shower, while on the road and at work too! What I didn't realise was that it was slowly seeping into my subconscious mind and it was beginning to take root until it became part of me. My habit of self-control was slowly being developed.

I also discovered that exercising self-control comes through practicing it day and night. The Lord showed me an image of an overweight person who was trying to get a six-pack, and that even though that person had the potential of developing that six-pack, he still needed to put in the work each day to have it. He said the person needed to watch what he ate, to exercise, sleep well, stress less and do abs exercises and that the person needed to be patient and consistent with the journey.

I knew what I had to do. I had the fruit of the spirit, but my walls were down, and they needed to be rebuilt. I had self-control but it was still a seedling that needed to be nurtured. This could only be done if it (self-control) were being exercised daily. I had the truth of God's word, so I began to work it out. Did I fail during the journey? Absolutely! I was like a baby who was trying to walk. My goal was to walk but I started out sitting, trying to crawl then I would fall back again. Once I crawled, I started attempting to stand then I'd fall again and again, but I refused to give up.

Another thing I did was that I asked for support. I asked my flatmate to look out for me whenever we would go out. I told my friends as well that I was on a weight loss journey. I woke up one morning and I decided to try walking. Was it easy? Yes, this time it was easy because God helped me each day and I also asked for help. Even though my flesh screamed from the new discipline it was facing each day I ignored it, silencing it by making declarations and I started gaining more ground with self-control.

Even now, I still guard my heart in this area. Often, I tell myself "Seun you have self-control in you, exercise it daily."

What Are The Steps I Took To Build Up My Wall And Exercise Self-control?

I've said this earlier on in this book, I made up my mind to lose weight. During my journey though, I realised I must have had an ulterior motive. So, I took time out to ask myself this question "Seun, why did you want to lose weight?'

My answer was this, I realised I didn't want to be emotionally ruled by food or circumstances anymore and I also wanted to leave a good legacy of divine health to my children. My reason for losing weight was not about me, I was no longer living for myself, my feelings and emotions. I was living for the next generation because from personal experience I knew being overweight as a child affected my self-confidence and led me to having low self-esteem. I did not want the generation after me to have such problems with their physical and emotional health.

Are you unsure why you want to lose weight? Tie it to something bigger than you because it sets your mind to look at the bigger picture when you feel tempted at times to quit, when you don't want to work out even though you know you should or when you don't want to eat a healthy meal. Let your reason be bigger than you. It made me want to exercise self-control on my journey and even when I fell at times, I got back up again. It was huge motivation for me.

Pay Attention To My Emotions: This was one of the most critical areas I had to work on and keep working on because I was an emotional eater by default (I used the word 'was' as I no longer identify with that person again). I had to watch what was going on in my mind most of the time. I started paying attention to my feelings, emotions, and moods each day and what I was exposing myself to. I found out through Joyce Meyer's book – Battlefield of the Mind, that I can choose my thoughts. I didn't have to allow or accept any thoughts that were not according to the will or word of God take root in me.

Do you know that what you hear, see, or feel affect your emotions daily? If you constantly hear you can do something, you will begin to feel or your emotions will be stirred up to want to do that thing; and so also if you hear every day that you can't do something, you will begin to believe that lie too and you will not be able to do it. Now I pay attention to my emotions. I feed my emotions with the word of God and when I am feeling down about something, I retrace my steps to find out how I got to that negative emotion and bring a correction straight away. For example, if I wake up feeling down for no apparent reason, I will go to the word of God and meditate on a scripture about joy or peace. I will say to myself "Seun the joy of the Lord is your strength." I might not feel that joy or peace straight away, but I know if I focus on it the emotion of sadness will soon turn into joy.

Why do I pay attention to my emotions? My emotions used to be the driving force of my life and I had to retrain them how to behave. God gave us good emotions like joy, peace, and love. Our emotions are ours to control and they can be very fickle, which means they are up one day and down the other. I learnt not to be moved by them but to be controlled by the spirit. Have you noticed that when you see a pair of shoes, for example, you get excited about them and buy them? After a few days, the excitement is gone, and you want something else that will bring that feeling of excitement. Paying attention to my good emotions and not focusing on the bad emotions helped me to build my walls. It didn't happen overnight but as I yielded to the spirit, I was able to rule and master it. Till now I still pay attention to my emotions.

Allocate Time To Exercise: This was one area I needed a lot of work on. It soon dawned on me that some challenges were easier to overcome than others. This is usually the case regarding any journey in life. I always thought exercise should happen if I felt like it. I didn't know it had to be planned for it to happen. I began to exercise self-control in this area.

I remembered how I gave up when I started exercising, calling my friend Bayo for a pity party and how she had called me to order saying 'Seun you are allowed to rest during your workout, but you must always finish whatever you start.' Well, that became my motto. Exercise had to be planned in advance in my case. I had to motivate myself and become my own cheerleader while my friend Bayo also supported me by keeping me accountable.

I realised that I couldn't rely on external motivation or inspiration. I basically took responsibility for my life. My default behaviour was to rely on my feelings so with the help of God, I started putting a plan in place. For example, I would ensure that I had my workout gear all planned on Sunday evening and know what exercise video I would be using in advance. It wasn't easy but was it worth it. I was steadfast taking it one day at a time! My workout time was my 'me time', time to reflect on my week and time to move and stretch my body.

I also found out that I would be reluctant and not always feel like working out but that feeling would only last for about five to ten minutes into the exercise. I quickly learnt not to rely on my feelings to move my body. Knowing the benefits of exercising the body also helped me to want to do it. The recommended physical activity for people between the ages of 18 – 60 years is 150 min (that's about two and a half hours) a day including strength training. If you want to lose weight you have to do about 300 minutes (five hours) a week.

Create Time: Time waits for no man. I had to also learn that you have to create time for certain activities. I used to think my meal prep or workout would just happen. When I had that mind-set, it didn't happen. When it did happen, it was based on whether I had time or not. I discovered that if I never created time to work out, the workout would not happen. I started creating time.

If for instance, I knew that in the coming week I was going to work out five days a week for 30 minutes, I would pick out my workout clothes the night before, leave them in the living room and put my laptop in a place that was easily accessible. I didn't realise that I was systematically creating a pattern in my mind. Thus, I'd wake up at 5 am – get out of bed and make a cup of green tea or warm water. I would spend some time praying, reading the word or listening to a message or a book. Then by 7 am I'd automatically get up and begin my work out. That saved me a lot of time. I remember before establishing this routine, whenever it was time to work out, I would stare at my wardrobe for about 15 minutes trying to decide what to wear. Meanwhile, time would be running out and before I knew it, I would start stressing myself out. So, one of the ways I was able to stop stress dominating my life was that I created time each day for my workout.

I am a morning person, so exercising in the evening was a 'no-no'! This didn't mean that I couldn't adapt if my circumstance changed and the need arose to change my pattern. I have learnt to be flexible with God no matter the situation. God is always the same today, yesterday, and forever, but our circumstances may change.

Allocate Time To Meal Prep: Meal prepping was work for me, I can't remember cooking that much growing up or during my university days. I lived on takeaway and I just didn't know any better. I had to quickly learn that for me to be successful on this journey I had to prepare my meals ahead of time.

The first thing I needed was to know how to cook. YouTube videos were a life saver! I would watch countless cooking videos and just go online to search for what I wanted to cook. Google became my friend and I used it daily. Most times, I would do a trial-and-error experiment but as I continued, I got better and better.

I realised also that I needed to have a food timetable. I would draw up a plan for the following week. For example, on a Friday or Saturday I would draw up a food timetable for Breakfast, Lunch and Dinner (it saved me lots of time and money). Then on Sunday night, which was normally my meal prep day, I would prepare my meals for four days at a stretch. So, if you asked me on a Monday morning what I would eat for breakfast on Wednesday morning or evening, I already knew. Building this structure into my life helped me to have a routine and structure and be in control.

Make A Shopping List: A shopping list is a list you make before you set out on your shopping expedition for food. The old me never really shopped or rather shopping for me back then was going into the store picking up pastries, biscuits, cakes, and fizzy drinks (well, I guess we can still call that shopping). I only knew a few aisles of the supermarket based on my shopping habits. I had never been through the fruits and vegetables aisle!

A shopping list was essential, it was a guide and it also helped me to navigate the stores very well. Once I had made my list before leaving the house, I was good to go. I would know which aisle to go and which one to avoid. I learnt to stock up on the staples like tinned beans, tinned fish, frozen vegetables or fruits, brown pasta or rice, frozen fish, or meat. It helped me to stay focused on my shopping trips and my shopping experience was smoother, faster, and enjoyable. Like I always say on my trips "If you don't want it in your basket, then don't stroll down the aisle." That slogan saved me lots of times and it prevented me from choosing the wrong food items.

Read Books: Reading didn't come to me naturally and this was because I never developed the habit while growing up. I didn't see the need to read but I learnt on my weight loss journey to invest time in reading books, it helped in personal development. I also happened to go to a church that had a reading culture, if you were to attend my church regularly you would develop a good reading habit.

At first it was difficult because I didn't know the benefits. However, I went on to purchase *Battlefield of the Mind* by Joyce Meyer, I learnt so much truth in that book and it transformed my life. After reading the book I made up my mind to become a reader. I started by reading Christian books, then I gradually moved on to reading books about personal development and my life took a 180-degree change. The change didn't happen overnight, but as I began to apply what I had read I started to see a positive change in my life. I was hooked.

God also used this newly developed habit to redirect my recreational outlet. Before my recreational time had been all about food and watching TV back-to-back, but now my life was being transformed by other people's success stories. The Bible says in **Proverbs 13: 20, NIV:**

"Walk with the wise and become wise, for a companion of fools suffers harm."

Since there was nobody for me to physically walk with, I chose to walk with the wise by reading their books. Now I enjoy reading, I can finish a book in two weeks depending on how big the book is. My weight loss journey transformed me into a reader. Don't underestimate what God will use your weight loss journey to do. He will do exceedingly and abundantly above what you could ever think of or ask for. Like I always say, you are not just losing weight, you are being transformed from the inside out if you allow God to use it for His glory.

Learning To Say 'No' To Others And 'Yes' To Myself: This was an extremely hard thing to conquer. I was once a 'people pleaser', I am no longer one. It was draining for me emotionally and psychically. I would commit to things that I had not thought through properly and leave more important personal matters to help others. Don't get me wrong, there is nothing wrong with helping others. I fell a victim to helping others while neglecting myself and it started to show in my life because I didn't allocate time to what mattered to me.

I overcame this by allocating time ahead for what I needed to do each day.

Whenever people asked me if I could do something for them and I knew it would either drain me emotionally or I wouldn't be able to attend to my own matters, I would always think it through and get back to them. In the past, I would have said yes without thinking things through but now through the help of the Holy Spirit, I have been able to come to that place of saying 'no' without feeling any guilt. For example, if a friend called me suddenly to attend a birthday celebration with her, I would say no especially if I knew it would interfere with a personal matter I had to attend to. However, if the same friend had given me four weeks' notice to attend a party with her, I might say yes because I know I can plan ahead.

One thing I have realised in life is that if you don't plan your time or life, people will plan it for you by demanding your time repeatedly. Saying no to so many distractions has given me focus which I needed not only on my weight loss journey but in life in general.

Set Your Mind: My mind like I said in the previous chapter was a wreck. I didn't know I could control it until I started seeing scriptures that talked about setting our minds on the right thing. The book of **Colossians 3: 2, NIV** says,

"Set your minds on things above, not on earthly things."

This means with the help of the Holy Spirit we can choose to set our mind on things that matter. Each day, I would set my mind on what I would eat or not eat ahead of time. One thing I struggled with in the beginning was discipline. I would eat whatever anyone offered me even though I packed my lunch. Once I had accepted this truth, I began to set my mind ahead of the day. My meal prep helped me because I would have planned what I would eat morning, afternoon, and night in advance. For example, if I got to work and someone was offering me a coke or a KFC meal, I would not think twice before saying 'no' because I had already set my mind and decided before I left home in the morning what I would eat during the day. On my way back from work, if the thought of grabbing chicken and chips came to mind, I would say to myself "You have dinner waiting at home for you, you don't need chicken and chips." As I did this, I began to recondition my mind to think a particular way each day and I began to experience total victory.

Prayer: My prayers were quite simple in the beginning of the journey – "Oh Lord I need your help, Lord help me. I can't do this without you. I am too weak to do this." They were simple and I knew God heard me, because each time I prayed my strength was renewed. Prayer for me meant asking God to help me on this journey daily, it meant I acknowledged that I didn't have the power on my own and I needed the supernatural power of God to help me.

I remember my pastor preaching about speaking in tongues and I began to practice it daily. The book of **Romans 8: 26-28, NIV** says,

> *"In the same way the Spirit [comes to us and] helps us in our weakness. We do not know what prayer to offer or how to offer it as we should, but the Spirit Himself [knows our need and at the right time] intercedes on our behalf with sighs and groanings too deep for words. And He who searches the hearts knows what the mind of the Spirit is, because the Spirit intercedes [before God] on behalf of God's people in accordance with God's will. And we know [with great confidence] that God [who is deeply concerned about us] causes all things to work together [as a plan] for good for those who love God, to those who are called according to His plan and purpose."*

Often during my prayer or quiet time with God, I would spend some time speaking in tongues to build myself up for the day.
The Bible tells us in the book of **Jude 1: 20, NIV,**

> *"But you, dear friends, build yourselves up in your most holy faith and pray in the Holy Spirit."*

I put the scripture above into practice and I soon found out that whenever I prayed in tongues during my quiet time or during any of my daily activities, the Lord gave me strength to get through the day. Often the Lord would give an interpretation of my prayers either by reminding me of a scripture or a book. Prayer for me was an empowerment during and after my weight loss. It was the source of my strength and ability to overcome emotional eating. Prayer works, start small and build up with God. God says in **Jeremiah 29: 12, NIV** says,

"Then you will call on me and come and pray to me, and I will listen to you."

God is a good Father; He wants and is always ready to do us good. This is the reason why when we approach Him in prayer at any time, He is willing to listen to us, guide us and answer our prayers in ways that are beyond our expectations. "He wants to set you free from emotional eating and other issues" praying was one of the ways I welcomed him in my journey, and even till now He takes all the glory.

Whenever people ask me how did you do it? I will always reply, "I was able to lose weight with the Lord's help."

Reminder: You have the seed of self-control, the fruit of the spirit in you. All you need to do is to acknowledge it first and begin to water it each day by using and exercising it over your situations and circumstances.

Plan of Action

The whole purpose of Book One is to get you thinking about your current lifestyle and how to begin to do the work that will get you to a more stable and healthier lifestyle.

1. What are the three most important areas that you really want to see a change? E.g. habits, mindset, or self-control.

a.
_____

b.
_____

c.

2. State below which one of the three is your top priority.

I commit to working on...

....

Remember you are making a commitment to yourself.

3. What plan have you put in place to achieve this goal?

4. What are the challenges or pitfalls that may stop you from achieving this goal?

5.What are the solutions you could use to overcome these challenges?

6.What support system do you have in place – friends, family, accountability *group, colleagues at work?*

7. I will review this goal on

....

Once you have achieved the first goal on your list, go and pick another one out of the top three and begin to work on it.

Change does not happen overnight. There is no button that's pushed to magically alter everything in your life. Change happens little by little, day by day, hour by hour, and minute by minute. Always remember with Christ you can do all things through Him who strengthens you.

Book
Two

Choices

You have the power to choose right, you just don't know it! When it comes to food, I really didn't know that I had the power within me (through the help of the Holy Spirit) to choose right daily. While growing up in an African home, you really don't have much choice when it comes to the food your parents give you daily. You must and will eat what they provide, whether it is healthy or not and may God help you if you don't finish everything on your plate! There's no debate about it.

I remember my mum serving me huge portions of food morning, afternoon, and night. I would eat my food and try to finish it even when I knew I would not be able to, it was forbidden in my home to leave any food on your plate. If you failed to complete your meal my mum would preach a whole sermon on how the poor people on the streets could only eat one meal a day and how fortunate we were to be able to afford three square meals.

This event from childhood marked me and I grew up thinking I didn't have a choice about what I could eat. I carried on with this habit for years and as a result I became overweight. On this journey, I learnt that I had the power to choose right daily and I had to exercise that power. The power of choice is just like that of self-control, you must exercise it daily.

In the beginning when God created man, he was given the power to choose right, it is called "will". God will not force a man to choose His way, which is always the best. He has given man the responsibility to exercise his will if man will acknowledge Him.

The book of **Deuteronomy 30: 19-20, NLT** says,

"Today I have given you the choice between life and death, between blessings

and curses. Now I call on heaven and earth to witness the choice you make. Oh, that you would choose life, so that you and your descendants might live! You can make this choice by loving the Lord your God, obeying him, and committing yourself firmly to him. This is the key to your life. And if you love and obey the Lord, you will live long in the land the Lord swore to give your ancestors Abraham, Isaac, and Jacob."

Can you see the power of choice that God has given us? The Bible in that passage uses the word *'today'*, it means each day of our life we have the power to choose right – the power to choose the right food, the power to choose to exercise even when you don't feel like it, the power to choose to say no to that cake or those biscuits when you are full, the power to set your mind on the right things throughout your day; and the more you exercise that power of choice the easier it becomes and you are able to gain victory on your weight loss journey.

What is the definition of 'choose'?

- To decide what you want from two or more things or possibilities.
- To think about which one of several things is the one you want, and take the action to get it.

From the definitions given above, we can see that choosing starts with either thinking or deciding between two or more things. Before my weight loss journey began, I never took the responsibility of deciding what was good to eat by myself. I often allowed the likes of McDonalds, KFC, Greggs, and other stores to decide for me each day. One thing I found out on my journey was that nobody was responsible for my health but me and only me. I was the one who had to daily take on the responsibility of choosing what I knew was good for my body. The moment I realised this, I quickly changed my perspective and started choosing wisely.

One thing I love about the human body is that it speaks to us and knows us, some people might not believe that; but whether we like it or not, our bodies give us signs to show how well we are taking care of them. When you constantly feel tired all the time or you feel bloated after eating certain food, it's a sign that your body is speaking to you. It is letting you know that the food you have just eaten is either good or bad for you. My body really helped me in the beginning to make better choices each day. I soon discovered that the more I fed it with healthy food, the more my moods stabilised, the dry patches under my armpits disappeared, the swelling of my breasts two weeks before my period stopped, and my period became less painful. These were some of the breakthroughs that enabled me to start making the right choices each day when I noticed the difference in the way I felt.

Each day I had to choose whether to meal prep or not and the more I meal prepped, the more I was able to control what went into my food, and I was able to save money. I chose meal prepping over buying junk food. I had to choose either to say no to cakes and pastries or say yes to fruits and nuts. The more I chose to eat fruits and nuts as snacks, the better I felt. Whenever I ate cakes or pastries, I would get a high sugar rush then come crashing down, and a few minutes after I had finished eating them, I would feel very sluggish.

I had to choose either to exercise or not each day. The more I chose to exercise, the more I had dopamine – the feel-good hormone. The good news is that with the help of the Holy Spirit, we can make healthy lifestyle choices each day and the more we make these choices, the stronger we become. You have the power to choose right based on the truth you know in Christ.

At times people ask me if I don't feel like eating certain foods like fried chips, cakes, biscuits, fizzy drinks, and my response to them is that I do feel like eating these foods at times (remember it is a feeling and by the grace of God I am no longer led by it). Yes, I do and that is the truth, but I don't yield or pay too much attention to these feelings. I have learnt not to allow my feelings to rule me but to allow my spirit man to be in charge. I often cite this example – if your manager annoys you at work and you feel like slapping him? Would you slap him or refrain from doing it? Of course, you would, even though you felt like slapping him you didn't because you know that there are consequences for slapping your manager – your immediate dismissal from work. The same also applies to me, I choose not to respond or rather, be led by my feelings. Over time with the help of the Holy Spirit, I have learnt not to respond to those feelings. It is just a feeling and it will go and if it doesn't, I might choose to pray about it or declare scriptures over myself and often the feelings leave.

Reminder: *With the help of the Holy Spirit living in you and leading you into all truth, you have the power to choose right based on your knowledge of the word of God. The more you know the word of God, the more you have the discernment and ability to choose right.*

Temptation

Temptation…I didn't even see it coming.

Maybe I should I say that the grace of God covered me from the beginning of my journey till the very end. Yes, His grace was there all along. A time came, however, when I was exposed to a variety of things on my journey. The first few months were quite smooth because I stopped buying junk food.

Before I embarked on my weight loss journey, I would normally have things like ice cream, cakes, and fizzy drinks at home. I remember hearing a quote once that says, "If you do not want to get into a fight you can't win, don't start it." I knew that if I had junk food in the house, I would be tempted. So, I immediately took control of my environment by ensuring I did not have any junk food around me, and I limited my access to it as much as possible.

Then I started another job and I felt I had been put into the lion's den to be devoured. What I didn't realise was that I had been put in that situation to test me and see if all I had learnt in the last few months about meal prepping, exercising, and choosing to exercise self-control had really left a positive mark on me. The truth is that you will be tested or tempted on this journey. These temptations have come to really prove what you believed or have learnt on your journey. So, relax, you will be fine because you have the Holy Spirit in you empowering you to say no to temptation. You should also know that God will always create a way of escape if or when you ask Him.

My weight loss journey with God was a process, and every single person who decides to lose weight will also go through a process on their journey. The result is that you will lose weight and become healthy. However, there are personal mind-sets and emotional trauma that God wants to deal with and heal you from, and it might take some time depending on whatever issues you might have. God knew that He needed to help me build a solid foundation on which my weight loss journey could stand, so the first few months were used to build things like knowing who I am in Christ Jesus, prayer, portion control, exercising, living beyond my feelings, choosing the right way of living, applying self-control, forming new habits, learning to say no to things that would normally lead to stress, and developing my emotional stability. The process was painful in the beginning, but in the end, it was worth it because I gained my freedom from emotional eating.

After a few months I had gotten a new job, I began another chapter and all I had learnt on my weight loss journey was tested. One thing I have learnt with God is that whatever you have learnt through the scriptures will always be tested to see whether you really know it or not.

I remember a particular day at work, even though I had prepared and brought a healthy meal with me for lunch, I had a huge craving to have something sweet and the thought lingered for a while, and it didn't go way. I knew something wasn't right and I just couldn't understand why I was feeling that way. After a few minutes at my desk, I cried out to God for help "Lord I really need your help, I don't know why I am having this sudden craving for something sweet." His reply was that I should take a walk. Taking a walk felt very silly, but I knew that whatever He told me to do would always work. I obeyed and stood up and took a walk for about ten minutes. By the time I got back to my desk the craving had gone. I felt very relieved, but I asked God again why I had such an intense craving, and His reply was this – you were bored! Isn't it surprising that something as insignificant as being bored can make you begin to crave sugary food? The mind doesn't like being idle!

The book of **1 Corinthians 10: 13, AMP** says,

> *"No temptation [regardless of its source] has overtaken or enticed you that is not common to human experience [nor is any temptation unusual or beyond human resistance]; but God is faithful [to His word—He is compassionate and trustworthy], and He will not let you be tempted beyond your ability [to resist], but along with the temptation He [has in the past and is now and] will [always] provide the way out as well, so that you will be able to endure it [without yielding, and will overcome temptation with joy]."*

This scripture really comforted me during my journey. It is often referenced when talking about being tempted to go back to fornication, pornography, or anger etc; but we can also apply the same scripture to weight loss.

One thing I have learnt about the word of God is that it has the answer to every single problem we have on earth; and that is why the word of God is the only solution to all human problems. There was no way I could have overcome that intense craving by my will power. Willpower will always fail because you are putting your confidence in your own ability and not God. The Bible says that we shouldn't put our confidence in the flesh, meaning do not even rely on it or even give it an inch in your life because the flesh is weak and dumb. It takes the spirit to subdue it and put it under the authority of God! I would have been defeated if I hadn't cried out to God when the cravings were intense, and He showed me a way of escape – taking a long walk.

After that incident, I went further to find out what the Bible says about temptation and how to overcome it because I knew this was a tip of the iceberg, and that many more temptations were yet to come. I needed to know how to deal with them on my weight loss journey.

The first thing I did was to do a Google search for scriptures on temptation and I began to read and study them. In the Garden of Eden, Eve was tempted and deceived by the devil. She and Adam had eaten the fruit that God had instructed them not to. Even Jesus was tempted after 40 days of fasting! Eve yielded to the temptation, while Jesus showed us the way to overcome temptation in this world.

This story of Jesus is the perfect example of how to not yield to temptation. So long as we are alive in this world, we will face temptation daily. The book of **Luke 17: 1, NIV** says,

> "One day Jesus said to his disciples, "There will always be temptations to sin, but what sorrow awaits the person who does the tempting."

Yes, that is the gospel truth but the good news for you and me, is that we have already overcome it. God is forever standing by to show us the way of escape when we ask Him to, and He will always show up.

The books of **Matthew 4: 1-11, NLT** says,

> "Then Jesus was led by the Spirit into the wilderness to be tempted there by the devil. For forty days and forty nights he fasted and became very hungry. During that time, the devil came and said to him, "If you are the Son of God, tell these stones to become loaves of bread." But Jesus told him, "No! The Scriptures say, 'People do not live by bread alone, but by every word that comes from the mouth of God.' Then the devil took him to the holy city, Jerusalem, to the highest point of the Temple, and said, "If you are the Son of God, jump off! For the Scriptures say, 'He will order his angels to protect you. And they will hold you up with their hands, so you won't even hurt your foot on a stone. Jesus responded, "The Scriptures also say, 'You must not test the Lord your God. Next the devil took him to the peak of a very high mountain and showed him all the kingdoms of the world and their glory. "I will give it all to you," he said, "if you will kneel down and worship me." "Get out of here, Satan," Jesus told him. "For the Scriptures say, 'You must worship the Lord

your God and serve only him. Then the devil went away, and angels came and took care of Jesus."

The Bible says Jesus was led by the spirit into the wilderness. We all know that the steps of a righteous man are ordered by God and we know Jesus knew God loved Him and wherever God lead Him would also be good, and He had the ability within Him to overcome the challenges. We all know what it feels like to be in the wilderness, in a place where it is dry, and nothing grows. Whether we like it or not, we will all experience a wilderness in one area of our life or the other, and that's where the devil came to Jesus to tempt him. The devil is very cunning and a deceiver. He waited for Jesus to be in a dry place and tempted Him after He had fasted for 40 days and 40 nights.

I learnt from studying this scripture that the devil will always tempt us when we are at our most vulnerable or when we are at our weakest. He is always looking for when our guard will be down to get in. Often, our guards are down when we are tired, stressed or under pressure, so watch out and be vigilant. **1 Peter 5: 8, AMP** says,

> *"Be sober [well balanced and self-disciplined], be alert and cautious at all times. That enemy of yours, the devil, prowls around like a roaring lion [fiercely hungry], seeking someone to devour. But resist him, be firm in your faith [against his attack—rooted, established, immovable], knowing that the same experiences of suffering are being experienced by your brothers and sisters throughout the world. [You do not suffer alone.]"*

I have experienced several situations like that. I seldom feel tempted because I now know what I need to do. When I find myself being tempted, I know I need to keep watch because it could either be, I am allowing stress into my life or I am not trusting God enough in a particular situation. For instance, I know that whenever I have an intense sugar craving, it could either be my period is on its way or I am bored, so I pay attention to my thoughts and get myself together by either praying or meditating on scriptures.

The Bible says the devil said to Jesus in **Matthew 4: 3-4, NLT,**

> *"If you are the Son of God, tell these stones to become loaves of bread." But Jesus told him, "No! The Scriptures say, 'People do not live by bread alone, but by every word that comes from the mouth of God."*

Can you see how the devil tried to play on Jesus identity first? He said, "if you are the son of God", of course we all know Jesus is the Son of God. The devil is very cunning and a deceiver, and he will constantly want to attack who we are in God first. For example, I know I can do all things through Christ who strengthens me, but I have been put in several situations where my flesh was telling me otherwise and it wanted to yield to the temptation. Thank God for the power of the word that has the ability to deliver. **2 Corinthians 10: 5, NKJV** says,

> *"Casting down arguments and every high thing that exalts itself against the knowledge of God, bringing every thought into captivity to the obedience of Christ."*

That's why Jesus told him,

> *"No! The Scriptures say, 'People do not live by bread alone, but by every word that comes from the mouth of God."* (**Matthew 4: 4, NLT**)

You can see how Jesus dealt with the temptations. He rebuked the devil using the word of God because that is the only word that the devil can resist. The devil will never bow down to just positive speech or talk. The only word that can keep him away and bring him to his knees is the word of God.

One thing that really made an impression on me was when Jesus said, "Man shall not live by bread alone but by every word that proceeds from the mouth of God." I had an 'Aha' moment that there are two types of food, one is the natural food we eat each day, and the other is the word of God which is spiritual food. It was then that it occurred to me that I can't just rely on natural food to live in this world, daily I have to also live by the word that proceeds from the month of the Lord daily! I needed the grace of God to do that. It was then I started drawing nearer to God as each day came, waiting during my quiet time to hear Him speak a word to me. I began to see the word of God as a *need* and not a *want*. I had to see it as a necessity. I needed it to live in this world as much as I needed my natural food.

1 Peter 2: 2, NASB says,

> *"Like new-born babies, long for the pure milk of the word, so that by it you may grow in respect to salvation."*

John 6:51, NASB says.

> *"I am the living bread that came down out of heaven; if anyone eats of this bread, he will live forever; and the bread also which I will give for the life of the world is My flesh."*

There are many more scriptures that talk about God's word being food, but I will limit it to this two above. The moment I had this awakening, spending time with God became a priority.

After the first temptation Jesus went on to face other temptations. Don't worry if you face temptations like this back-to-back, I did too on my journey and I still face them from time to time. The important thing is knowing and doing what Jesus did to defeat the enemy. The Bible says

> *"The devil departed from him for a season"* (**Luke 4:13, KJV**)

Once the devil sees that you have become stronger in a place, he will leave you alone for a while and will keep looking for another opportunity to tempt you again. The Bible says the devil goes around like a roaring lion, looking for whom to devour. He is powerless but he will always come behaving 'like' a roaring lion meaning he is not one (a lion), but he is always looking for someone to devour(destroy).

became very vigilant during my journey and even after all these years I am still vigilant. The story of Jesus being tempted in the wilderness, and how He overcame each temptation is a perfect example of how God wants us to respond to any temptation that comes our way. Through Christ Jesus we have overcome the power of the enemy over us and we have what it takes within us to stand against any temptation on any journey in life (including weight loss) if we ask God for help each time. I still humble myself each time I face temptation to ask God for help. He always shows me an escape route.

have talked about temptation and how God will always show us a way to overcome it. Let us now look at how to identify hunger and how to identify a craving. I must admit, I didn't know how to identify either one of them because it seemed as if I was hungry all the time. One of the main reasons for this was that I was eating processed food most of the time (cakes and pastries, which don't fill you up for long). As soon as I started training my body to eat the right food each day, I began to pay attention to what hunger and cravings felt like because I discovered I was experiencing a lot of cravings. What I didn't know was that cravings are often caused by external and internal triggers. External triggers are what you see, touch, smell, taste and hear. External triggers always work with our five senses as mentioned above. Examples include the smell of freshly baked bread or pastries, seeing a TV advert about some certain type of food you like, seeing others eating in front of you, walking past one of your favourite takeaways shops like a fish and chips shop, McDonalds, KFC etc. All things that affect your five senses and cause you to act are external triggers. Internal triggers, on the other hand, are thoughts, feelings, hunger, and cravings.

Hunger is a physiological need. It is our body's way of telling us it needs fuel. I didn't know this at the beginning of my journey, so I had to learn it. Hunger will not disappear if you are truly hungry, this sensation will only continue to grow. Hunger tends to be general – you would eat pretty much any food if it were offered.

Cravings are an intense psychological desire to eat a particular type of food, even if you are not hungry. Cravings will tend to diminish, if not go completely if you distract yourself for 20 – 30minutes. Cravings are specific – typically for sweet, fatty, salty foods. Since I wanted to be free from emotional eating, I had to know the difference between the two (hunger and craving). It has been a lifesaver for me. Knowing how to identify the difference has helped me overcome emotional eating. I found out that the times I often experienced intense craving was when was stressed, bored, discouraged, celebrating or joyful. Cravings come with a mix of emotions and once I was able to identify them and follow the process of waiting 20 to 30 minutes by either distracting myself by taking a long walk, drinking water, reading a book, I knew it would pass. If it didn't pass after 30 minutes, then I knew it was hunger I was dealing with. I realised that cravings come like a wave and they come with a desire to eat a particular type of food which is either salty, fatty, or sweet.

The table below can help us identify what a craving or hunger is like in our daily lives

Hunger And Craving Table

You missed breakfast and by mid – morning feel ravenous	Hunger
You are having a pint or coke at the pub and see crisps behind the bar which makes you feel like eating	Craving
You finish a large meal and feel like something sweet	Craving
Your stomach starts to rumble just before lunch	Hunger

You are at a football match and the smell of hot chips makes you feel like eating	Craving
You are doing the grocery shopping and there is a 1-2-1 offer on chocolate bars or plantains chips which makes you feel like eating	Craving
Someone in the tearoom at work is talking about cake and you feel like eating	Craving
You haven't thought about eating today and are starting to get the shakes	Hunger
You fill up your car at the petrol station and the sight of sweets at the till makes you feel like eating more	Craving
Your colleague at work offers you half of their sandwich, which then makes you feel like eating more	Both
You feel lightheaded as a consequence of not eating all afternoon	Hunger
You are always starving at a certain time of day	Both

The table is really an eye opener to help us see where we are going wrong and what we can do when either a craving or hunger comes. Cravings will come, but it is what we do when they come that help us overcome them.

Reminder: *You have what it takes in you to overcome temptation on your journey, don't fret or be timid when it comes, ask the Holy Spirit to help you and you will find a way of escape.*

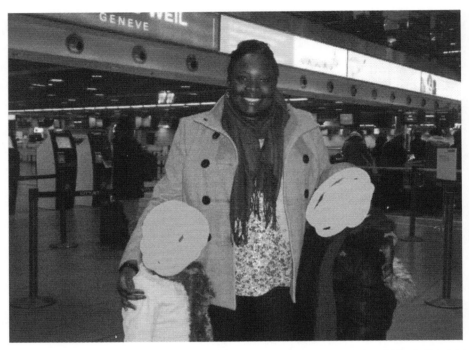

What Is On My Plate – Then And Now?

"Let food be thy medicine, and let medicine be thy food"

This saying above is often ascribed to Hippocrates (400 BC), and used to emphasise the importance of nutrition in preventing or curing disease. Yes, this is so true. All the natural foods we eat have been created by God to give our body daily nourishment, to be enjoyed and also to give us energy to carry out our God given purposes on earth. One of the first things God did when He created man in the beginning was to show him what He had already planned and created for him to feed his body with daily. **Genesis 1: 29-30, NLT** says,

> *"Then God said, "**Look! I have given you every seed-bearing plant throughout the earth and all the fruit trees for your food.** And I have given every green plant as food for all the wild animals, the birds in the sky, and the small animals that scurry along the ground—everything that has life." And that is what happened."*

God is such a master planner that even when He made man, He also took the responsibility to provide for man and showed him what he needed to feed his body, and not only did He care about man, but he also took it further to create food for the animals. Isn't our Heavenly Father caring and nurturing to ensure everything He created is provided for properly?

The food I use to eat was causing death to my body. I was constantly bloated. My period was hell on earth, my breasts were always sore and heavy two weeks before my period and two weeks after my period I would be back to being bloated again. My sugar cravings during my periods were out of control. I would have dark patches under my armpits and on my neck all the time. I constantly felt tired and very sluggish. I had very bad back pains all the time and I felt very heavy when moving around.

Looking back now, I was just a mindless and emotional eater, I didn't pay attention to what I ate or the portion control (I didn't even know that I was meant to portion control my food). I felt my body wasn't my own, but I still kept on, eating all the wrong food until I decided to lose weight.

About six to nine months into my weight loss journey, almost every single symptom I complained of had reduce significantly or disappeared. It felt like a dream. I went from being bloated to not being bloated. My breasts were no longer sore. The dark patches I use to have were gone. The tiredness and sluggishness that overwhelmed me went away, the back pain disappeared, the mood swings disappeared, the sugar cravings were gone, the depression and anxiety vanished; and I felt like a brand-new person. All of this happened as a result of making daily changes to what I ate, what I heard and what I saw.

I have heard thousands of testimonies from people who saw a radical change in their health when they decided to lose weight or chose to live a much healthier lifestyle, testimonies of PCOS (Polycystic Ovary Syndrome), irregular periods or no period at all, back pains, insomnia, depression and anxiety, osteoarthritis, sleep apnoea, migraines, high cholesterol, Type 2 diabetes, all gone. These people generally feel better because they chose to change their eating habits.

One thing that really helped me was that I was open to change. I really and truly was ready to change my eating habits and I took baby steps towards it each day. I felt my body was given another chance to live again after all the years I had fed it with the wrong food.

My old ways of eating are no longer a part of me. I had been a glutton. Friends have told me that they were shocked at the amount of food I use to put on my plate. Below is a table showing how I used to eat.

Old Food Timetable

	Mon.	Tue.	Wed.	Thurs.	Fri.	Sat.	Sun.
Breakfast	3 croissants and a cup of hot chocolate with sugar	1 large hot chocolate drink with sugar and two muffins	1 beef pie from Greggs/ Percy Ingle with a 500ml bottle of coke	3 croissants and a cup of hot chocolate with sugar	1 large pie from Greggs with a 500ml bottle of coke	Cold 500ml bottle of coke	No meal
Lunch	KFC 2 pieces meal (2 fried chicken), 1 large chips, baked beans, 1 large coke	Nando's 1 quarter chicken with chips and rice and unlimited coke	Eat as much as you like Chinese's takeaway with McDonald's milkshake	Tuna sweetcorn baguette with a bottle of Lucozade	Nando's 1 quarter chicken with chips and rice and unlimited coke	Biscuits or cake bought from the store with a bottle of Lucozade	Large portion of white rice with fried beef stew (takeaway)
Dinner	A large portion of Jollof rice with chicken and a 500ml Bottle of coke	Large portion of white rice with fried beef stew (takeaway) and a bottle of Lucozade drink	Large portion of fish and chips with 500ml bottle of coke	Agege bread with butter and a cup of cold hot chocolate drink	Large digestive biscuits with 500ml of coke.	Agege bread with butter and a cup of cold hot chocolate drink	Large Rich Tea biscuits with 500ml of coke.

Just by looking at this food timetable you can see that I didn't drink water. I lived on at least to three to four bottles of coke and Lucozade a day, with countless cups of hot chocolate. My go to snacks were always doughnuts, cakes, salted or sugary nuts, or biscuits. The only time I remember drinking water was having it as an ingredient when making a cup of hot chocolate. You can also see that most of my meals were fried. I don't recollect cooking much. I lived on takeaway all the time, and most of the time the takeaway food was fried.

- Breakfast – Pastries from Greggs or Percy Ingle, croissants, cakes, and biscuits.
- Lunch – Takeaway Chinese, Nando's, Fried chips and chicken or fish or sausages.
- Dinner – White rice with stew, chicken and chips or fish, cakes, meat pie, puff Agege bread with butter or sardines
- Drinks – Fizzy drinks of all kinds – Coke, Fanta, sprite, Lucozade, or any fizzy

drink on offer.

• Snacks – Cakes, biscuits, salted nuts, sweets, and chocolate.

I can't remember ever cooking. 98% of my food was store bought and not cooked by me. I really didn't know how I survived eating like that. My body was aching and dying slowly each day. I was constantly tired, irritated, and moody. My life was full of worry and anxiety. I noticed that as I began to clean up my eating habits, the symptoms above disappeared each day. My body was healing itself with the new healthy food I was eating each day.

Could the illness or tiredness you feel each day be due to the type of food you eat? Could your irritability or moodiness be a consequence of the junk food you eat? Could your unstable emotions be linked to what you eat each day?

The more I paid attention to what I was putting into my mouth combined with studying and knowing the word of God more, I could see the cloud of depression was being lifted each day.

The research below will give you more insight to how what we eat can be linked to depression and anxiety.

Research 1

Eating junk food raises risk of depression, says multi-country study - Analysis of 41 studies leads to calls for GPs to give dietary advice as part of treatment.

Eating junk food increases the risk of becoming depressed, a study has found, prompting calls for doctors to routinely give dietary advice to patients as part of their treatment for depression.

In contrast, those who follow a traditional Mediterranean diet are much less likely to develop depression because the fish, fruit, nuts, and vegetables that diet involves help protect against Britain's commonest mental health problem, the research suggests. Published in the journal **Molecular Psychiatry,** the findings have come from an analysis by researchers from Britain, Spain and Australia who examined 41 previous studies on the links between diet and depression.

"A pro-inflammatory diet can induce systemic inflammation, and this can directly increase the risk for depression," said Dr Camille Lassale, the study's lead author. Bad diet heightens the risk of depression to a significant extent, she added. The analysis found that foods containing a lot of fat or sugar, or was processed, lead to inflammation of not just the gut but the whole body, known as "systemic inflammation". In that respect the impact of poor diet is like that of smoking, pollution, obesity, and lack of exercise. "Chronic inflammation can affect mental health by transporting pro-inflammatory molecules into the brain it can also affect the molecules – neurotransmitters – responsible for mood regulation," said Lassale, who is based at the Department of Epidemiology and Public Health at University College London.

The research showed that poor diet has a likely causal link with the onset of depression and not merely an association. They did not find that their result were explained by people who are depressed eating more poor-quality food, or that they were depressed to start with, she stressed. They based their conclusion on reviewing five longitudinal studies of 32,908 adults from the UK, France Spain, Australia, and the US. "Poor diet may increase the risk of depression a these are results from longitudinal studies which excluded people with depression at the beginning of the study. Therefore, the studies looked at how diet at baseline is related to new cases of depression," Lassale said.

One in six adults in the UK are thought to experience depression, often alongside anxiety. The Centre for Mental Health think-tank has estimated the illness overall cost to society, including lost productivity as well as NHS treatment, is £105bn a year. Dr Tasnime Akbaraly, another UCL academic who co-authored the research, said: "Added to recent randomised trials showing beneficial effects of dietary improvement on depression outcomes, there are now strong arguments in favour of regarding diet as mainstream in psychiatric medicine. "Our study findings support routine dietary counselling as part of a doctor's office visit, especially with mental health practitioners." Dr Cosmo Hallstrom, a depression expert and fellow of the Royal College of Psychiatrists, said that if junk food did raise the risk of depression then an unhealthy diet was not just bad for the body but also the mind. "The chemistry in the gut is very similar to the chemistry in the brain. So, it's not surprising that things that influence the gut might influence the brain too," he added. Prof Helen Stokes-Lampard, the chair of the Royal College of GPs, said: "This large-scale study provides further supportive evidence that eating a healthy diet can improve our mood and help give us more energy. It adds to the growing body of research which shows that what we eat may have an impact on our mental health. "Increasingly, more GPs are recommending that their patients try to make sensible diet and lifestyle changes as part of a holistic approach to the management of chronic diseases because we know it may have a range of a positive effects on our patients' physical and mental health."

Research 2

Junk food diet raises depression risk, researchers find by - Manchester Metropolitan University

A diet of fast food, cakes and processed meat increases your risk of depression, according to researchers at Manchester Metropolitan University. A paper from Manchester Metropolitan's Bioscience Research Centre found that eating a diet containing foods which are known to promote inflammation – such as those high in cholesterol, saturated fats and carbohydrates – makes you around 40% more likely to develop depression.

The researchers analysed data from 11 existing studies that focused on the link between depression and pro-inflammatory diets – encompassing more than 100,000 participants of varied age (16-72 years old), gender and ethnicity, spanning the USA, Australia, Europe and the Middle East. All the studies recorded the presence of depression or depressive symptoms in the participants (through self-observation, medical diagnoses and/or antidepressant use), alongside a detailed questionnaire about the contents of their diet.

Each participant was assigned a score of how inflammatory his or her diet is, according to the dietary inflammatory index. Some of the studies were cross-sectional, using data that was immediately available, and other studies tracked participants for up to 13 years. Across all studies, participants who had a more pro-inflammatory diet were, on average, 1.4 times more likely to have depression or depressive symptoms. The results were consistent regardless of age or gender – and were the same over both short and long follow-up periods. Dr Steven Bradburn is from the Bioscience Research Centre at Manchester Metropolitan's School of Healthcare Science. He said:

> "These results have tremendous clinical potential for the treatment of depression, and if it holds true, other diseases such as Alzheimer's which also have an underlying inflammatory component."

Simply changing what we eat may be a cheaper alternative to pharmacological interventions, which often come with side-effects. "This work builds on recent advances in the field by others, including the first ever clinical trial into dietary interventions for treating depression, which have shown beneficial improvements in depressive symptoms. It should be stressed, however, that our findings are an association, rather than causality. Further work is needed to confirm the efficacy of modulating dietary patterns in treating depression with relation to inflammation."

An anti-inflammatory diet—containing more fibre, vitamins (especially A, C, D) and unsaturated fats—has the opposite effect and could be implemented as a treatment for depression. Therefore, a Mediterranean diet of olive oil, tomatoes, green vegetables and fatty fish could help lower depressive symptoms. Inflammation is the body's natural defence system against infections, injuries and toxins. In order to protect itself from harm, the body releases proteins, antibodies and increased blood-flow to affected areas, causing redness and swelling. However, chronic inflammation puts the body in a constant state of alert and has previously been linked to diseases such as cancer, asthma and heart disease. Such persistent inflammation, particularly in the brain, is believed to contribute to neuronal death. The research, 'An anti-inflammatory diet as a potential intervention for depressive disorders: A systematic review and meta-analysis', is published in *Clinical Nutrition.*

The research above gives you a balanced idea of how depression and what we eat are linked. I didn't follow the Mediterranean diet discussed in the research above.

I believe it would be fair to say that what we eat contributes to how we feel, our moods, our emotions, and our outlook to life a lot of the time. Once you know that and begin to make a change, then your transformation to a healthy you start.

I noticed that the food I ate each day, affected my emotions and mood. I realised that when I ate a healthy breakfast, I felt stable, focused and alert throughout the day. I wouldn't get irritated over things and I was quick to let go of so many things. I believe a lot of us are always thinking of what we will lose on this journey, rather than what we will gain. What I gained can't be compared to what I lost. I gained life and experienced real life. I gained my self-confidence back, my health back, my prayer life back, my body back and my mind back.

The Eatwell Plate guide on the NHS website was a lifesaver for me. What I did was to tailor it work for me. Living healthy is a lifestyle and you need to lay the foundation with the right eating patterns, so that you can keep to it for life. Can you live on eggs, fat, and little vegetables for life? Can you live without eating carbs for life? Can you live without eating sugar for life? Can you live without frying your food for life? You have to be decisive and with the help of God, He will instruct you on what way to eat and how to go about it. Therefore, losing weight is a personal journey to everyone, it is a calling to something greater that you, it is a call to living the rich and satisfying life Christ came to give you!

The truth is that I am not against any diet or way of eating. What I would recommend is a change of lifestyle (habits or behaviours) or eating habits. The diet industry is full of mysteries, and if you are not careful you will be deceived easily and misled with so many 30 days challenges or quick transformation pictures – "I lost 20 lbs. in 1 month" (yes, they work but that is just the starting point). It is a multimillion-pound industry that feeds from people's lack of patience and people who want a quick fix. The average person doesn't want to put in the work to lose weight. Losing weight and staying healthy will demand you being intentional daily, focused, consistent, committed, persevering, getting knowledgeable, applying acts of self-love and self-care, persistence, discipline, patience, building habits over a long period of time, refusing to give up, letting go of worry and anxiety, stress and above all, letting God be in control. It takes someone who is relentless and has made up his/her mind to see the journey to the end. That person could be you if you ask God for help and don't give up. Anyone can lose weight once they make up their mind to do so. Like I always say, losing weight is the starting point, but maintaining a new and healthy weight is the real work. You can do this once you have established a pattern of building ong lasting habits.

So, with all the changes above that I have made, what is or what does my plate look like now? The Eatwell Plate was a guide for me and really helped with portion control and knowing what my plate ought to look like. I started off by following the Eatwell Plate, but I later tailored it to what suited me which I call 'Balance Plate'. It was easy to follow with my main meal. I knew counting calories would stress me out and I was prone to being easily addicted, so God guided me by leading me to two simple ways that worked for me. This has been my way/pattern of eating for the last nine years.

God knows you better than you know yourself. He created your body; He knows your personality and He is the only one that can give you wisdom regarding what type of eating habits you should follow. He will guide you and lead you each minute at a time, each day at a time, each meal at a time, each setback at a time, and each victory at a time till you get to the end of the journey.

Below we will find out what the Eatwell Plate is all about and how it can help us to feed our body well.

The Eatwell Plate

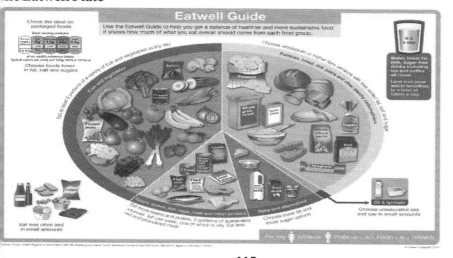

The Department of Health, England's Eatwell Guide is the UK's healthy eating model. It is a simple, practical tool to help us make healthy choices and to show the proportions in which different food groups are needed to make up a healthy balanced diet.

Is The Eatwell Guide For You?

The Eatwell Guide applies to most people regardless of weight, dietary restrictions/ preferences, or ethnic origin. However, it doesn't apply to children under two because they have different nutritional needs. Between the ages of two and five, children should gradually move to eating the same foods as the rest of the family, in the proportions shown on the Eatwell Guide. Anyone with special dietary requirements or medical needs might want to check with a registered dietician on how to adapt the Eatwell Guide to meet their individual needs.

How Can The Eatwell Guide Help?

The Eatwell Guide shows the different types of foods and drinks we should consume and in what proportions to have a healthy, balanced diet. The Eatwell Guide shows the proportions of the main food groups that form a healthy balanced diet:

- Eat at least five portions of a variety of fruit and vegetables each day.
- Base meals on potatoes, bread, rice, pasta, or other starchy carbohydrates choosing whole grain or wholemeal versions.
- Have some dairy or dairy alternatives (such as soya drinks), choosing lower fat and lower sugar options.
- Eat some beans, pulses, fish, eggs, meat, and other proteins (including two portions of fish, every week, one of which should be oily)
- Choose unsaturated oils and spreads and eat in small amounts
- Drink 6-8 cups/glasses of fluid a day if consuming foods and drinks high in fat, salt, or sugar, have these less often and in small amounts.

The eat well guide plate can be use whenever you are deciding what to eat, a home cooking, out shopping for groceries, eating out in a restaurant, café, or canteen etc.

How Does It Work?

The Eatwell Guide divides the foods and drinks we consume into five main groups. Try to choose a variety of different foods from each of the groups to help you get the wide range of nutrients your body needs to stay healthy and work properly. It is important to get some fat in the diet, however, foods high in fat, salt and sugar are placed outside of the main image as these types of foods are not essential in the diet, and most of us need to cut down on these to achieve our healthy balance. Unsaturated fats from plant sources, for example vegetable oil or olive oil, are healthier types of fat. Remember, all types of fat are high in energy and so should only be eaten in small amounts.

Let us take a closer look at each of the food groups.

Fruit and Vegetables

Most of us know that we should be eating more fruit and vegetables, but many of us aren't eating enough. Fruit and vegetables should make up just over a third of the food we eat each day. Aim to eat at least five portions of a variety of fruit and vegetables each day. If you count how many portions you're having, it might help you increase the amount and variety of fruit and vegetables you eat. Choose from fresh and frozen. A portion is 80g or any of these: 1 apple, banana, pear, orange or other similar-size fruit, three heaped tablespoons of vegetables, a dessert bowl of salad, 30g of dried fruit (which should be kept to mealtimes) or a 150ml glass of fruit juice or smoothie (counts as a maximum of one portion a day).

Potatoes, Bread, Rice, Pasta and Other Starchy Carbohydrates

Starchy food is an important part of a healthy diet and should make up just over a third of the food we eat. Choose higher-fibre, wholegrain varieties when you can by purchasing whole-wheat pasta, brown rice, or simply leaving the skins on potatoes. Base your meals around starchy carbohydrate foods. So, you could:

- Start the day with a wholegrain breakfast cereal; choose one lower in salt and sugars.
- Have a sandwich for lunch.
- Round off the day with potatoes, pasta, or rice as a base for your evening meal.

Why choose wholegrain? Wholegrain food contains more fibre than white or refined starchy food, and often more of other nutrients. We also digest wholegrain food more slowly so it can help us feel full for a longer period. Wholegrain food includes wholemeal and wholegrain bread, pitta and chapatti, whole-wheat pasta, brown rice, wholegrain breakfast cereals and whole oats.

Dairy and Alternatives

Try to have some milk and dairy food (or dairy alternatives) – such as cheese, yoghurt etc. These are good sources of protein and vitamins, and they are also an important source of calcium, which helps to keep our bones strong. Some dairy food can be high in fat and saturated fat, but there are plenty of lower-fat options to choose from. Go for lower fat and lower sugar products where possible. For example, why not try 1% fat milk which contains about half the fat of semi-skimmed milk without a noticeable change in taste or texture? Or you can try reduced fat cheese which is also widely available. Or you could have just a smaller amount of the full-fat varieties less often. When buying dairy alternatives, go for unsweetened, calcium-fortified versions.

Beans, Pulses, Fish, Eggs, Meat and Other Proteins

These foods are sources of protein, vitamins, and minerals, so it is important to eat some foods from this group. Beans, peas, and lentils (which are all types of pulses) are good alternatives to meat because they are naturally very low in fat, and they are high in fibre, protein, vitamins and minerals. Pulses, or legumes as they are sometimes called, are edible seeds that grow in pods and include foods like lentils, chickpeas, beans, and peas. Other vegetable-based sources of protein include tofu, bean all of which are widely available in most retailers. Aim for at least two portions (2 x 140g) of fish a week, including a portion of oily fish. Most people should be eating more fish, but there are recommended limits for oily fish, crab, and some types of white fish. Some types of meat are high in fat, particularly saturated fat. So, when you're buying meat, remember that the type of cut or meat product you choose, and how you cook it, can make a big difference. To cut down on fat: choose lean cuts of meat and go for leaner mince, cut the fat off meat and the skin off chicken, try to grill meat and fish instead of frying and have a boiled or poached egg instead of fried.

Oils and Spreads

Although some fat in the diet is essential, generally we are eating too much saturated fat and need to reduce our consumption. Unsaturated fats are healthier fats that are usually from plant sources and in liquid form as oil, for example vegetable oil, rapeseed oil and olive oil. Swapping to unsaturated fats will help to reduce cholesterol in the blood, therefore it is important to get most of our fat from unsaturated oils. Choosing lower fat spreads, as opposed to butter, is a good way to reduce your saturated fat intake. Remember that all types of fat are high in energy and should be limited in the diet.

Foods High In Fat, Salt and Sugars

This includes products such as chocolate, cakes, biscuits, full-sugar soft drinks, butter, and ice-cream. These foods are not needed in the diet and so, if included, should only be done infrequently and in small amounts. If you consume these foods and drinks often, try to limit their consumption so you have them less often and in smaller amounts. Food and drinks high in fat and sugar contain lots of energy, particularly when you have large servings. Check the label and avoid foods which are high in fat, salt and sugar.

Hydration – Aim to drink 6-8 glasses of fluid every day

Water and sugar-free drinks including tea and coffee all count. Sugary drinks are one of the main contributors to excess sugar consumption amongst children and adults in the UK. Swap sugary soft drinks for water. Alcohol also contains lots of calories (kcal) and should be limited to no more than 14 units (this is equivalent to six pints of beer or seven glasses of wine) per week for men and women. The calorific content of an alcoholic beverage depends on the type of alcohol, the volume served and the addition of mixers.

What we have discussed above is what the Eatwell guide is all about. They all played a major part on my weight loss journey and they will continually play a part on this journey of having and living a healthy life. Losing weight is 80% food and 20% exercise, consequently I spent a lot of my time reading, studying on the impact of the above and healthy eating in general, during and after my journey. According to the Momenta philosophy, and based on their studies, exercise and a healthy diet play a huge role in what leads to long term weight loss. Momenta is a global weight management specialist company based in the UK. These studies found that out of 5000 people, who have lost a large amount of weight: 89% used both a healthy diet and exercise to lose weight, 10% used just diet and 1% used just exercise. On my journey, I used the combination of a healthy diet and exercise to change my lifestyle and it is still very much a part of me.

After studying the Eatwell Plate, knowing what food group I needed to eat often and what my plate should look like at each mealtime, I knew following it daily would be a struggle for me because of the nature of food we Africans eat. I searched further online to find how to make each one of my meals look simpler. With the help and guidance of God, I came upon what I call the Balance Plate. What a life saver! This was what I needed, something simple and straight forward that would require me to eat a balanced meal.

The Balance Plate

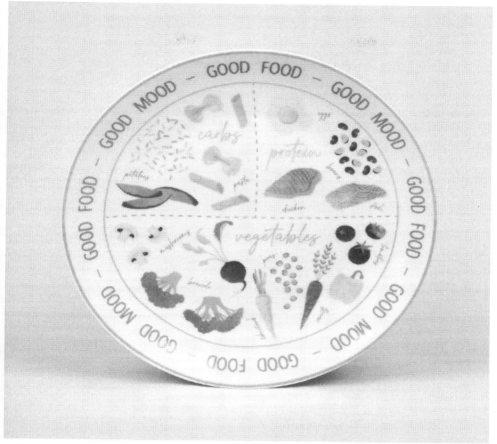

website: www.matalan.co.uk

What is a Balance Plate?

The Balance Plate model according to Momenta, is a simple tool designed by experts to help you divide up your plate at main mealtimes. It is a simple way to get a healthy mix of nutrients, control your portion sizes and stay fuller for longer. Experts advise that

- Half of your plate should be composed of vegetables (broccoli, cauliflower, green beans, carrot, lettuce, cucumber, cabbage, mixed salad, mixed veg, vegetable soup etc).
- A quarter of your plate should be composed of starches (potatoes, sweet potatoes, brown rice, wild rice, whole – wheat pasta, whole wheat couscous, quinoa, bulgur wheat, bean pudding). When it comes to how I would portion my swallow, I had to use my fist as a measure of eba, amala and iyan (popular Nigerian meals which I often eat).
- A quarter of your plate should be composed of meat or its alternatives (lean meat or chicken or turkey, fish, egg, and tofu.

In my research I stumbled across this plate. I wasn't ready to count calories and I was looking for something proven and easy to use to help me manage portion control (my portion sizes before I started my weight loss had been ridiculous). This worked very well for me, but I still had to take baby steps and be consistent about it. How could I, a girl whose plate was often half filled with refined carbs become a girl who now filled half of her plate with vegetables, and the remaining half filled with a combination of carbs and protein? Initially it was hard because I had to retrain my mind and my appetite to start eating this way. Did I stay the course even though I felt like giving up? Yes, I did. I've said it before, I took it one day at a time and after two weeks it became much easier.

In the last few years, I have recommended this plate to people who don't know how to start their weight loss journey or even reduce their portions, and the feedback has been amazing. Even as a Momenta weight loss coach, I find myself often referring to this way of eating because it works and it is so easy to follow and guess what? You will see the weight drop off over a long period of time if you stick with it. Always remember whatever way you decide to eat will work if you are willing to do the work and stick with it.

Reminder: *You can retrain your taste buds to love healthy and real food, it will take a while for the change to happen. Keep choosing healthy food each second, minute, hour, and day; and one day you will wake up and find out that it (healthy food) is what your body will be asking for. Change is possible if you don't give up and are open to it.*

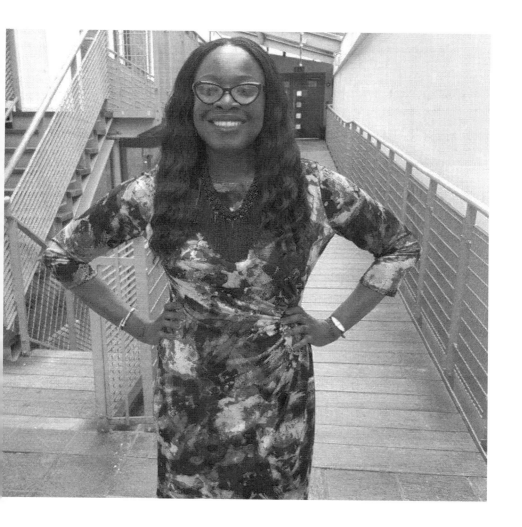

Supernatural Provision

My God shall supply all my needs according to his riches in Christ Jesus
(Philippians 4: 19)

What a journey (of self-discovery and weight loss) I had to go through by faith! I was brought up in a Christian home, but I didn't become born again until I was about 14 years old. The memory of that day is still so much alive in me (when I gave my life to Jesus). Although it was a voluntary decision I made, I went back to my old ways of living and just never really committed to the new life in Christ Jesus.

Life continued, I left secondary school, went to the university, and finally moved to the UK for study. I was still a Christian – I went to church on Sundays, joined the evangelism team (I was very zealous in it), attended the Wednesday prayer meetings and just did everything in the natural I believed a Christian should do. If I needed to know what the next step to take in my life was, I would go and meet a pastor or a prophet to pray for me and reveal God's plans for me. That was how I lived for years.

In the year 2009, I began to have a longing to know God much better, but I ignored this feeling and carried on with my life.

Then the big church I attended was asked to leave their old building, which they did. As a result of this move, two churches emerged. I made the decision to stay with the smaller church because I believed God was calling me to build a relationship with Him. During all of that, I was made redundant at my place of work and my whole life came crashing down, I was in a CRISIS. Everything I had built my hopes on crumbled. I had never been out of work before, so I didn't know how to handle the circumstances I found myself in. God knew all of this was coming and it was why He had put that longing in me to know Him more. I am grateful now that I made that decision to follow that instinct.

I had joined the smaller church, but I was still one leg in and one leg out. It was hard for me to break the habit of looking for a perpetual intermediary (someone who would hear God for me) between me and God. I felt like someone who had been eating meat and leeks (in Egypt like the children of Israelite), and suddenly, I was required to start a new diet of manna (something unknown that I'd never eaten before). I told the Lord I was not prepared to eat manna and that I wouldn't!

I was still going to the new church every Sunday. On these Sundays, the Pastor would ask for a volunteer to stand up and read the Bible study hand-out for the week. I would never offer my services, I always remained seated. Most of the time it was because I was suffering from the aftereffects of having gone out to a party the night before. I always had one event or the other I would attend each weekend. I was a partygoer! From one owambe (party) to the other, birthday parties, baby showers and naming ceremonies, I would be there. Even when I didn't receive an invitation, I was willing and happy to tag along. I was never at home. Sitting down at home seemed very strange to me then. Nowadays, I happily stay at home. I don't need to go out to seek amusement and enjoyment. The good news was that despite my eventful Saturdays, somehow, I still always made it to church each Sunday.

During this period, I was still relying on my savings to carry me through until I could get another job. I went for interviews back-to-back and nothing happened. By this time, I became worried, anxious, and depressed (at the time I didn't know I was going through depression, I was down). It started gradually and it built with time. I didn't feel like going out anymore, the zeal for life was beginning to wane, my outlook on life was hopeless and pressure from my parents to find a life partner was mounting; and I could no longer hide the feelings of low self-esteem and lack of confidence I had covered up for years. I believe this was part of what led to my suicidal thoughts. I began to hear voices daily, they were strange and weird telling me "Nobody cares about you", "Why don't you just give up, after all you will not be missed?", "Can't you see all that your parents want you to do is get married and make them proud?", "Can't you see that nobody wants or needs you?", "The last person you dated dumped you and got married to someone else within six months", "Is life worth living? Have you even achieved any of the goals you set for yourself in life?"

I felt like a total failure at that point in my life, my insecurities and low self-esteem began to lead me down a dark path of no return. I had friends around me, but I didn't give them a clue as to what I was thinking or what I was about to do. On the outside I looked all well put together, but on the inside, I was dying. I have met people from all walks of life that had experienced feelings of hopelessness like I did in the past, and one thing we all agreed upon is feeling that sense of hopelessness and not seeing a way out of our circumstances in life.

What made my case worse at that time, was that I was not entitled to government benefits or universal credit based on my UK settlement. I was in a tight corner and a hopeless situation. What next? Where could I go? Who would help me out? Who would supernaturally supply me? Well, I had come to the end of myself and there was nowhere to turn to. What did I do next? I didn't have a choice but to look up to God, but this time around it was different for me compared to before when I would seek him through a pastor or prophet.

I remember one Sunday, I got to church early, and I paid attention to the Bible study, then came the Sunday message. I remember the pastor talking that morning about how God wants and desires to have an intimate relationship with us, how God wants us to trust Him with our lives, the decisions we make and the choices we make. He also talked about how God has a purpose for our lives, that He didn't just put us on this earth to work our 9-5 jobs, and that God has a specific assignment for everyone and also how God has already made daily provisions for us. Somehow, for the first time in my life, all that got my attention (God has a great sense of humour right) and I thought I will give this relationship thing with God a try. After church I met with the pastor to tell him that I was ready to have an intimate relationship with God and ask him what I should do next. I remember he told me to start reading the gospels. I also told him I was hearing voices every now again, telling me to give up on life and commit suicide. He prayed for me, speaking the word of God into my life and started checking up on me daily to see how I was doing (this was almost nine years ago when mental health issues were not as talked about as they are now). I am thankful that I didn't have to go down the road of anti-depressant medication or go through another way out.

Please hear me out, God has a different route for each person's recovery (to make you whole) and if the path He is leading you to is a talking therapy or taking medication, please do it until He gives you the next direction. God has already paid the price to set you free based on what Jesus did for you and me on the cross, He wants you to enjoy freedom in your health – mind and body.

John 3:16, NIV says,

> *"For God so loved the world that he gave his one and only Son, that whoever believes in him shall not perish but have eternal life."*

You can see from this scripture just how much you are loved by the Father and the reason why He gave Jesus Christ (the best thing He had) to us all is so that we will not perish, meaning that He doesn't want us to experience death in any area of our life including our mind and health.

In my own case, I needed to know who I was in Christ. It was the foundation that needed to be laid for my freedom from mental health illness and to also enable me deal with some soul issues, i.e., my self-worth problems – lack of self-esteem or self-confidence, unforgiveness and worries about life. I was glad God did amazing work in me as I began to develop an intimate relationship with Him.

Knowing who you are in Christ is a foundational truth we all need to be established in, and a necessity for every Christian because until you know who you are, you will not live a victorious life on earth. We are constantly in a spiritual battle whether we feel it or not. The Bible tells us in **Ephesians 6: 10,** who we are to fight, what type of weapons God has supplied for us to fight with in this battle, and what part we are to take. I discovered that you cannot deal with a soul problem (I talk about the spirit, soul, and body in the chapters ahead) by just taking a pill or talking to a therapist. A pill cannot address and heal you of emotional trauma. You need understanding, revelation or insight from the word of God; and you need to accept the truth you have seen from the word then consistently, apply it until it becomes your reality or your new normal (I've discussed this process earlier which I called the renewing of the mind according to **Romans 12: 2**). For me, taking a pill would never have solved the problems of not feeling loved, not feeling good enough or the of feelings of rejection since childhood, jumping from one relationship to the other, not knowing how to make better choices or even knowing why God created me. It was only the love of my Heavenly Father that could heal those wounds deeply embedded in my soul. God did amazing things for me over a period as I spent more and more time getting to know Him through His word.

The word of God is living and powerful, it cleanses our hearts, it is a light and a lamp, it makes you whole, it restores, it shows you your potential and reveals God's intentional plan for your life, it heals, it shows you the mind of God concerning you, it defines you, it sets you free, it makes the impossible possible, it creates new things out of nothing, it makes you brand new and it puts you in right standing with God. There is nothing in this world that the word cannot recreate or restore. The world we live in answers and submits to the word of God. We should not forget that the world was created and framed by the word of God according to **Hebrews 11:2** and the book of **Genesis 1 & 2.**

I have said this before, it wasn't easy for me in the beginning. It was a slow and steady process with many stumbling blocks along the way. I dedicated time each morning to reading the Bible, and a lot of the time I found it boring. God helped by prompting me to reach out to my pastor who encouraged and advised me (he was always gracious to me and constantly built me up with the word of God). After God used him to intervene, the same word which I had claimed was boring and confusing started ministering life to me, the experience was out of this world. God communicated with me through His word, speaking to my circumstances, reassuring me that I was loved, that He was going to turn things around, that He had not left me nor forsaken me.

I remember reading the story of Elijah in the book of **1 Kings 17:1-7, NJKV**
> *"And Elijah the Tishbite, of the inhabitants of Gilead, said to Ahab, "As the Lord God of Israel lives, before whom I stand, there shall not be dew nor rain these years, except at my word." Then the word of the Lord came to him, saying, "Get away from here and turn eastward, and hide by the Brook Cherith, which flows into the Jordan. And it will be that you shall drink from the brook, and I have commanded the ravens to feed you there." So, he went and did according to the word of the Lord, for he went and stayed by the Brook Cherith, which flows into the Jordan. The ravens brought him bread and meat in the morning, and bread and meat in the evening; and he drank from the brook. And it happened after a while that the brook dried up, because there had been no rain in the land.*

When I read that scripture, I believed that God was going to send help to me, and it would be in an unusual way. I also believed He was telling me to stay in the UK because I had been thinking of moving back to Nigeria. 'Stay by the brook' for me meant stay in the UK and 'ravens brought him meat and bread' was that God would provide for me in an unusual way. I needed to believe this 'impossibility', I didn't have a choice, and this was God teaching me personally how to walk by faith and not by sight.

A few days later a long-time friend came in from Nigeria and asked if we could meet up. At first, I was reluctant, but I remembered that I wasn't working so I didn't really have anything to lose by meeting up with him. What I didn't know was that the friend was actually the 'raven' God was sending from afar to surprise me (we can never beat God at supplying His children, if He needs to raise someone from another country, He will do it). I met up with my friend, but I never told him I was job hunting. When I was about to leave, he surprised me by handing me a £100 note. I collected the money, and, on my way home, the Lord ministered to me that, what He had shown me in the Word was coming to pass. I screamed and I thanked Him. This was I who in the past had thought I could never hear from God. The Lord was teaching me how to walk by faith and not by sight, it was mind blowing! The word of God tells us how we as Christians were designed to live in **Romans 1: 17, NKJV:**

> *"For in it the righteousness of God is revealed from faith to faith; as it is written, "The just shall live by faith."*

The just here means a believer or a disciple of Christ should live his/her daily life by faith which is being guided by the written word of God.

This led me to the question – what is faith?

The book of **Hebrews 11: 1-2, NKJV** says,

> *"Now faith is the substance of things hoped for, the evidence of things not seen. For by it the elders obtained a good testimony."*

So how did I get this faith? **Romans 10: 17, NKJV** says,

> *"So, then faith comes by hearing, and hearing by the word of God."*

The more I spent time reading the word of God, my faith in God and what I needed to trust Him for was growing daily, and the ability to hear from Him was becoming clearer too.

A few weeks later, I received a letter from Her Majesty's Revenue & Customs (HMRC) informing me that I had overpaid a tax to the tune of about £250! I had been out of work for about nine months, so how did I overpay tax? My tax code was still the same from before I lost my job. I called HMRC and they confirmed that they did indeed owe me a tax refund. What surprised me even more was that I received almost £1000 from HMRC that year. The cheques kept coming every two months. I felt like I was living in a dream. All this had happened just by believing that God would take care of my needs. My bank also sent me a cheque of about £80 saying they had mistakenly charged me for an overdraft. I was overwhelmed with God's favour during that period of my life, it felt unreal, but God showed me that He would take care of me if only I allowed Him no matter what my circumstances looked like in the natural. I learnt how to walk by faith just by following the word of God as He said it.

While He was supernaturally providing in the natural, He was also healing my soul. Each day I dove into the Bible, read it, meditated on His words, asking questions, showed up at prayer meetings, and started reading books that encouraged spiritual growth. The thoughts and heaviness of worry, lack of joy, depression and suicide began to fade. It didn't happen overnight but the more I spent time with God, the less I heard those voices of hopelessness, and instead the voice of peace from God that surpasses all human understanding began to flood my heart. Praise God!

For over a period of nine months I dedicated myself to the word of God and one day I discovered that depression and suicidal thoughts had completely disappeared never. I received my freedom in Christ.

I have to emphasise the fact that I was ready to change and confront my issues which was very important for my journey of healing. Anyone who wants to embark upon a journey of healing too has to accept that fact. Healing can be messy at times because God through His word will unpeel layers of issues to get to the foundation. There were days I just wanted to give up because it was easier to blame God and others for my issues. Healing with God made me take responsibility for my life, it exposed my excuses, it exposed the things I found comfort in; and it stripped me of the old image of myself and began to build a new image in me. God is a healer. **Psalm 107: 20, NKJV** says,

> *"He sent His word and healed them and delivered them from their destructions."*

Nobody can heal you like God can, when He finishes with you, you will feel like a brand-new creation (which you already are in Christ). The book of **John 8: 32, NKJV** says,

> *"And you shall know the truth, and the truth shall make you free."*

You shall know the truth, which is God's word, and the truth you know shall set you free. Do you want to be free? Know the truth, accept the truth, abide in the truth, and stand on the truth. Despite everything that had happened, I vividly remember crying to God one day about my rent being overdue and the Lord told me through the book of **Ruth 2: 9, NKJV:**

> *"Let your eyes be on the field which they reap and go after them. Have I not commanded the young men not to touch you?"*

As I read the book and came across this verse, I knew what the Lord was saying.

He had commanded my flatmate not to ask me for rent till I started work again and guess what, she never asked me or put pressure on me during that period. I knew at that time that it had become important for me to see the word of God as a necessity, it is one of His various means of communicating with us daily. Most days I followed through by reading the word even if nothing seemed to stand out to me from what I had read. I learned to discipline myself by spending time with Him even when life issues happened at times, I would always ensure that I studied God's word irrespective of my feelings in the moment.

Miraculously, my church also started giving me welfare money. That really helped and a very good friend of mine helped me out too. I never asked any of these people for help, but God used them to bless me when I needed it. There are many examples I could give. I remember one Sunday, £250 was left in the middle of my Bible and I did not find out until I received a text from the donor to check my Bible. The £250 came in as a miracle, on that day all I had left on me was £10. I had made up my mind that I would top up my oyster card to ensure that I could get to church and come back home; and I would give the remainder of £5 as an offering. I didn't know that God had a bigger and a better plan for me, He had touched the heart of someone in church to give me money.

Another time I received £1200 from someone who told me that God put it in their heart to give me for the process of my naturalisation in the UK. I remember praying to God about it and just leaving it in His hands. Quite a few people I knew at the time had qualified for theirs and were applying. My case was hugely different, I was not working. What gave me the boldness to even think I could go ahead and ask God for money to apply? I had built and grown my faith over a period, so it was very easy for me to ask God to do what seemed impossible. I remember asking people who had applied, and they all told me I didn't measure up because I wasn't working, and I would need to provide a six to twelve weeks' pay slip. Furthermore, it would take about six months to hear back from the

Home Office. I was paralysed with fear, but I believed since God had supplied the money then He would make a way out. I learnt during this period to be careful who I asked for advice. God in His mercy prompted me to share the testimony of the money for my naturalisation with my pastor who then asked me if I had applied, I told him no. He asked why, I told him I wasn't working and that there was a requirement explicitly stated on the form that I had to submit it with six to twelve-month payslip. He immediately said it was not so and that if I checked the form carefully what was required was either a payslip or a P45 or P60 (details of Employee Leaving Work Tax Form or End of Year Certificate Tax Form) and, I could back it up with a letter with proof that I was looking for a job. God used my pastor to open my eyes. I did this and sent my application through and I remember declaring one morning that my application would be approved within six weeks and not six months as others had experienced. To the glory of God, my application was approved and returned within four weeks.

God used the experiences above to show me that I didn't have to believe or rely on other people's experience. He wanted me to be careful who I shared things with and once He told me to do something, I should believe Him totally. There were different occasions that I can't explain when I would receive £50 or more just when I needed to sort out my essentials. God took good care of me in that season, I experienced supernatural provision. I learnt to walk by faith and not by sight. I learnt to know and hear the voice of God for myself. God used that time to start the good work of learning to trust, lean and rely on Him for everything. It was during this period that I got the strength to lose weight! Isn't God amazing?

All this happened because I woke up one morning and realised that I couldn't continue living my life as I once had and I needed to rely totally on God, and He was there for me. What the enemy meant for evil, to kill and destroy me, God used it to bring out a transformation in me and that birthed this book. I am writing this part of the book to show you that God heals, God makes whole, and

God still supplies needs supernaturally regardless of natural circumstances. The God we serve can be trusted with our lives and he will never leave us nor forsake us. **Philippians 4: 19, NKJV** says,

"And my God shall supply all your need according to His riches in glory by Christ Jesus."

Paul says 'my God' meaning he knew and had experienced this God he was talking about and 'shall' not maybe, meaning it is a certainty. He will supply all your needs and yes that means financial, physical, emotional, and spiritual needs! They are all covered according to His riches in glory in Christ Jesus, not according to your bank accounts or the systems of provision in this world. Let my story stir up your faith to trust God for the supernatural.

Reminder: *He that began a good work in you will complete. God will supply all your needs and not just some if you will lean and rely on Him. If He needs to send someone from another country to fulfil a need in your life, He will send that person speedily. Be encouraged and open your heart to Him, be ready to be wowed by your Heavenly Father.*

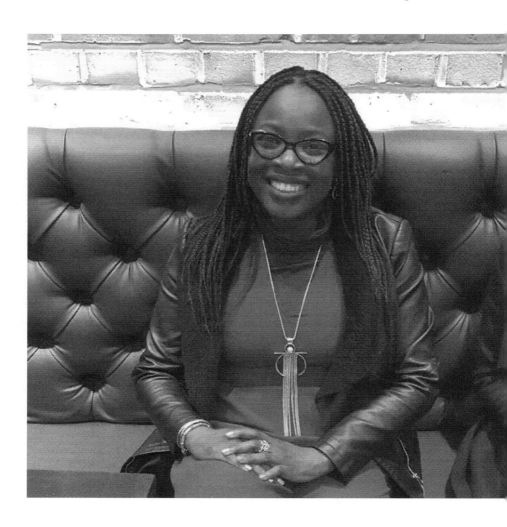

2017

It Is A Lifestyle, Not A Diet

From dealing with the root causes of emotional eating to finding a way when all odds were against me, to forming new habits, to overcoming temptation, to applying self-control daily, to knowing how to choose my thoughts on a day to day basis, to portion controlling my food, to reading food labels and decluttering my house; to the glory of God, I lost over 35kgs or 66 pounds within 1.5 years, and I have by the grace of God been able to maintain it for the last nine years. I went from a size 42DD Marks & Spencer (M&S) bra size to 34G and from a dress size of 22 to a size 12. This is the reason I say, God took me on a journey of self-discovery. He used this weight loss journey to show me what I can do with His help and guidance on how through His grace I could overcome overeating and any other issues life may bring.

Now I can truly say that a lasting weight loss journey must be a lifestyle change (knowing who you are, renewing your mind, choosing positive thoughts daily, guarding your heart daily, forming new behaviour, managing your emotional triggers, exercising self-control, knowing your external triggers, being led by God daily etc) which starts from the inside out. A diet only addresses your outer body struggles and not your inner life or mind, and it is not lasting. Real change, the God kind of change, happens on the inside out and it is lasting and permanent. God used this journey to build me from the inside out.

What is a Lifestyle?
It is a way of living of individuals, families (households), and societies, which they manifest in coping with their physical, psychological, social, and economic environments on a day-to-day basis.

The **Cambridge** Dictionary defines the word *'lifestyle'* as a particular way a person or group lives and the values and ideas supported by that person or group or someone's way of living.

We can see from the definition above that a lifestyle is a way of living by choice. When you decide to lose weight, you are deciding to change from your old ways of living to start a new way of living. Losing weight is a lifestyle change and not a diet. When you consistently change your way of living, it becomes a habit, and it becomes a lifestyle forever. Nobody arrives there in a day, it's all about taking it one step at a time or one day at a time.

I am sure by now, you are probably thinking "Seun, I want the same result that you had, and I believe God can do the same thing for me. How do I start this lifestyle change to lose weight or change my attitude about my health? What can I do to permanently change from yo-yo dieting to finally losing weight and keeping it off? How do I discover the real me?"

The truth is that one answer does not fit all. God has a personalised plan for you regarding your weight loss journey and He is already waiting on you to call upon Him to help you and guide you on this journey. What works for Miss A will not work for Mrs B, what works for Mr G will not work for Mr Y. The important thing is that you ask God to show you, which way He has mapped out for you and then follow it till the end.

Practical Steps To Take To Embark On Your Weight Loss Journey With God

The God Factor: My weight loss journey started and finished with God. Frequently when people ask me, how did you lose weight? My reply is "God helped me" or I will say, "I lost weight with the help of God." Often people are shocked because they have never thought of asking God for help when it comes to losing weight. My relationship with God was at the core of my successful weight loss journey. Like I said earlier, I was weak physically, emotionally, spiritually, and financially and I could only ever overcome it all through my intimate relationship with Him. God made us for relationship and that is the core of the book of **Genesis 1 and 2**. Adam had a wonderful relationship with God in the beginning, he fellowshipped with God day and night. Adam had access to God 24/7 in the Garden of Eden until the devil came in to tempt Eve and that was where man lost that relationship, and sin and separation entered the world. The good news was Jesus came to restore that relationship back by paying the price for our sin on the cross and by restoring us to our wonderful relationship with our father. All sins forgiven, all debts paid and just by what Jesus did we were made a new creation (brand new). God is our Heavenly Father, He created and formed each one of us for His glory and each day, He is longing to hear from us to fellowship with Him.

The book of John 3:16, NKJV says,

"For God so loved the world that He gave His only begotten Son, that whoever believes in Him should not perish but have everlasting life.

Ephesians 2: 1-10, NIV says,

"As for you, you were dead in your transgressions and sins, in which you used to live when you followed the ways of this world and of the ruler of the kingdom of the air, the spirit who is now at work in those who are disobedient. All of us also lived among them at one time, gratifying the cravings of our flesh and following its desires and thoughts. Like the rest, we were by nature deserving of wrath. But because of his great love for us, God, who is rich in mercy, made us alive with Christ even when we were dead in transgressions—it is by grace you have been saved. And God raised us up with Christ and seated us with him in the heavenly realms in Christ Jesus, in order that in the coming ages he might show the incomparable riches of his grace, expressed in his kindness to us in Christ Jesus. For it is by grace you have been saved, through faith—and this is not from yourselves, it is the gift of God—not

by works, so that no one can boast. For we are God's handiwork, created in
Christ Jesus to do good works, which God prepared in advance for us to do."

You can see through the scriptures above what happened at redemption! So, get
God involved on your journey, He knows where the real issues (for me – lack of
confidence, low self-esteem, bitterness, unforgiveness, rejection, mindless
eating, laziness, always giving excuses, emotional eating, lack of portion control
etc) are and He is able and willing to work with you to overcome those issues.
The Bible says in the book of **John 15: 5, NLT,**

   "Yes, I am the vine; you are the branches. Those who remain in me, and I in
   them, will produce much fruit. For apart from me you can do nothing!"

That is the truth! Apart from Him you can't experience lasting change or victory
on your weight loss journey or lifestyle change. From today, get Him involved by
building a relationship with Him. Spend time in the place of prayer and tell Him
how you need His help daily. Spend time reading and studying the Bible,
meditate on His word daily, listen to messages online that will transform your
soul. God is good and He can't wait to help you every single step of the day.

It Starts with the Mind: The human mind is one of our greatest investment. Your
mind is priceless. Whatever you think in your mind you can become. There is no
limit to how far you can go in life if you harness the power of the mind. Your
mind has the creative ability to see and create the impossible and that is how God
designed it to function. The devil knows this very well, so every day he is looking
for ways to ensure you don't harness the power in your mind, hence the worry,
anxiety and pressures of this world, all have been designed by him to hack your
mind. The Bible says according to the book of **Proverbs 23:7, NKJV** as a man
thinks in his heart so is he. You can never rise above the level of your thoughts.
Our thoughts are the driving seats of our life. If you believe you cannot, then you
cannot if you believe you can, so you will.

One area the Lord led me to work on continuously was my thoughts. My thought life was a junk house, I believed what anybody or my circumstances said about my life. As I began to have an intimate relationship with God, I began to see that I needed to align my thoughts with Godly thoughts daily. Was it easy? No. Did I take it one day at time? Yes. The truth is that we must continually renew our mind with the word of God I had to go through a renovation of my thoughts during and after my journey. I once believed I would never amount to anything in life, I once believed I was worth nothing, I once believed I was of no significance. Even as I'm writing all these things that I once believed, I laugh now because I now know the truth in God's word, and it is this truth that sets me free. I now know I am loved, precious and honourable, worthy, a special treasure, God's own possession, uncommon, a new creation, righteous, redeemed, and great!

The book of Roman 12: 2, NLT says,

> *"Don't copy the behaviour and customs of this world, but let God transform you into a new person by changing the way you think. Then you will learn to know God's will for you, which is good and pleasing and perfect."*

The scripture above tells us that we can change the way we think with the help of the Holy Spirit, if we want to and the only way to prove God's will for our life is to change our thinking daily to align with the way God thinks which we can learn through His word. The renewing of the mind is a process, it doesn't happen overnight but by faith you can begin to follow this principle and see your weight loss journey progress, or any other area of your life transformed. Little by little, you can take back your mind by renewing it with the word of God. For example, if you are struggling with losing weight and you have lost faith in your ability to do so based on the unsuccessful attempts you have made in the past or based on feelings of being overwhelmed when you started or you just can't seem to follow up till the end; you can start by mediating on these scriptures below.

Philippians 4: 13, NKJV

> *"I can do all things through Christ who strengthens me."*

2 Timothy 1: 7, NIV

"For the Spirit God gave us does not make us timid, but gives us power, love and self-discipline."

Isaiah 41: 10, NIV

"So do not fear, for I am with you; do not be dismayed, for I am your God. I will strengthen you and help you; I will uphold you with my righteous right hand."

Ephesians 3: 16, NIV

"I pray that out of his glorious riches he may strengthen you with power through his Spirit in your inner being."

Meditate on these passages before you go to bed, do the same thing when you wake up, before going to the gym or during your workout. Say them to yourself repeatedly. As you do this, you are reprogramming your mind and after a while you will see that what looked overwhelming or impossible is possible based on the truth in those scriptures. Whatever God tells you to do, He supplies the strength to do it and yes, you can lose weight through Christ who strengthens you. Remember it is not your strength but the strength of Christ who lives in you.

Prayer: Prayer is the key, no matter how simple it is. In fact, the simpler it is the better it is. I believe prayer is communicating with God daily and just simply humbling ourselves before Him and trusting by faith that He hears us, and He will answer us according to His will. Since we know He hears us when we make our requests, we also know that He will give us what we ask for (**1 John 5: 15, NLT**).

Many people in the Bible offered prayers to God in their time of need and God answered them in different ways. I remember when I started my journey, my prayers were very simple like "God I need your help. Lord I don't know what to do each day" and He began to lead me, nudging me little by little. I humbled myself daily in the place of prayer and He show up with much grace and wisdom. The Bible says in the book of **James 4: 6, NLT:**

> *"And he gives grace generously. As the Scriptures say, "God opposes the proud but gives grace to the humble."*

Each day, I humbled myself in the place of prayer and asked for help on what to do and He always answered.

As you begin to do this, please pay attention to the thoughts or pictures that come to your mind throughout the day because He will begin to give you answers this way most of the time.

I remembered when I was confused about what workout to do, I prayed about it and while having my bath, I had a thought to call my friend Bayo for help and I immediately followed through; and that was how my prayer was answered with that problem.

Prayer is key and knowing that your Heavenly Father can't wait to hear from you each morning is so reassuring and knowing that He is our present help in time of need is also comforting. Ask in prayer and God will show you a way out.

Know Who You Are In Christ: This is one truth you will have to know and keep working on until you are well-rooted and established in it. One of the many reasons behind my weight issue was not knowing who I was in Christ. Basically, I had an identity issue, and I did not love who I was. I struggled with knowing I was loved, accepted, beautiful, treasured, precious and chosen; and all of this drove me to food for comfort. I can't remember my dad ever telling me "Seun I love you" or "Seun you are beautiful." The first time I heard the phrase "I love you" was from the mouth of my first boyfriend. I had never known or experienced the love of my dad, so I began to seek love from other sources and I inevitably made the wrong choices in relationships.

On my journey, knowing that God loves me unconditionally was the beginning of the healing of my soul. I had never felt loved before. I always sought the acceptance and approval of my parents through my accomplishments in life, but it never worked. They constantly compared me with other people and the thought of never being good enough clouded my judgement when it came to matters about myself. It was a back-to-back battle until I realised that God my Heavenly Father, the one who created me and knew me before He formed me in my mother's womb, loved me unconditionally; and saw me as His special treasure and His possession. It was an eye opener for me and that was what I needed to know and hear repeatedly to begin the healing of my soul.

The truth above didn't transform me immediately, but as I kept beholding the truth in God's words day and night, the renewal of my mind was happening, and I was becoming rooted in it. Now I know from the bottom of my heart and through the scriptures that no matter what my circumstances appear to be or what my feelings are telling me, or what sin I may have committed, God loves me deeply and unconditionally, and He alone has a good plan for my life.

Even with all these revelations, I still must actively guard my heart against any attack of the enemy. Till today I still meditate on some scriptures like the ones given below.

Romans 5: 8, NLT

"But God showed his great love for us by sending Christ to die for us while we were still sinners."

John 3: 16, TPT

"For this is how much God loved the world—he gave his one and only, unique Son as a gift. So now everyone who believes in him will never perish but experience everlasting life."

Be Open to Change: Nothing happens in our comfort zone, meaning nothing happens if you choose not to be open to change. Many people want to lose weight, but they are not ready to give up their old ways of living to adapt to a new way of living or even pay the price. You can't lose weight without being open to change and the truth is that change can be difficult and painful at the same time, but it will always yield a great result if you choose not to give up on the journey. Most of the successful people we see in the world went through a similar process and that is why we hear about them today.

Let me use myself as an example, I was stuck in my old ways of just eating vegetables occasionally, but on my journey, I discovered that if I needed to get to my desired weight loss goal, I needed to give up my old way of eating and adapt to a new way of eating. I did this but the change in my body didn't happen immediately. However, with a lot of persistence and patience I soon began to see the benefits of eating a variety of vegetables, like having good bowel movement, an increase in the vitamins and nutrients my body needed, feeling less bloated and many more. Was it painful? Yes. Was it worth it? Yes.

The word of God says it very plainly according in **Hebrews 12: 11, NIV** that

"No discipline seems pleasant at the time, but painful. Later, however, it produces a harvest of righteousness and peace for those who have been trained by it."

Discipline for me in my case meant coming out of my comfort zone, saying no to junk food, getting out of bed to exercise in the morning, saying no to stress, meal prepping, saving money, being selfless, not giving into negative emotions etc.

Afterwards though there was a sense of peace and right living that had emerged because of this discipline.

The pain of changing is worth it because after the change you will produce a harvest of righteousness (the right way of living) and peace. It is worth all the sweat and pain. Abraham, in the Bible, was called out of his comfort zone when he had to leave his father's house, his country and his relatives to go to the land God would show him. Moses was called out of his comfort zone when he had to lead the children of Israel out of Egypt. Gideon was called out of his comfort zone when he had to save the children of Israel from the Midianites. Ruth came out of her comfort zone and followed Naomi her mother-in-law to a land where she had no family, to seek prosperity in the land for both.

When you are being led by God on any journey of life, you will be called out of your comfort zone to experience something bigger and better for you. By coming out of your comfort zone, God will begin to empower you supernaturally to do what you can't do for yourself. Each one of the people in the Bible mentioned above, took one step without seeing the next step. Make up your mind by trusting God that you will do that exercise even if you don't know where the strength will come from. You might need to choose to eat that vegetable and start drinking water by faith, trusting God to change your appetite as you do your part. I have learnt from my weight loss journey to be open to change in life and the only things constant in life are God and change. Please remember that there is enough grace to carry you through that principle of change. Let me also leave you with some quotes on change.

"A mind is like a parachute. It doesn't work if it is not open."
-Frank Zappa

"It's only after you've stepped outside your comfort zone that you begin to

change, grow, and transform."
- **Roy T. Bennett**

"You never change your life until you step out of your comfort zone; change begins at the end of your comfort zone."
-**Roy T. Bennett**

Know Your 'Why': It is important you know your 'why.' It is important that you know the reason why you want to lose weight, get out of debt etc. So, ask yourself "Why do I want to lose weight?", "Why do I want to get out of debt?", "Am I doing it for myself, my kids or my husband?"

I knew my 'why' when I started. I didn't want to be an emotional eater any longer. That is the reason why God did work in my soul and at the same time my body. I knew I was an emotional eater and I no longer wanted to live my life being led by my emotions all the time. This was what motivated me on those days my feelings were all over the place. That 'why' was what motivated me when I felt like giving up several times. I had to remind myself daily why I was on this weight loss journey and as I progressed, the 'why' began to change (it will change from time to time). My why moved from not wanting to be an emotional eater, to now wanting to be healthy to fulfil my purpose of being a healthy mother to my children.

Your 'why' could be getting into a size 10, 12 or 14 dress, for others that 'why' could be being able to wear that bikini at the beach or being able to fit onto that ride on the playground, or the seat in an aeroplane. Our reasons will be different, don't worry if it doesn't look like someone else's, and God is very pleased with that because He has different journeys planned out for everyone.

Once you have established your 'why', then remind yourself daily about it by writing it down somewhere or putting it up somewhere you can constantly see it. You can also tell your spouse, family, friends, and colleagues at work, to remind you of your 'why'. The Holy Spirit, above all, is very good at reminding us too. Once your why is established, you can also do something that is visual to remind you why you are doing what you are doing, because you will need it for days when you feel like giving up (you will have days like that, but you can overcome them).

Go to the Root Cause: Going to the root cause just simply means knowing how you got to where you are today with your weight gain. Was your weight gain from childhood? Did you suffer trauma that led to you being an emotional eater? Was your weight gain triggered by the loss of a family member? Was it triggered by the loss of a job or a partner? Was it because you were a mindless eater? Was it because you just had a baby? Was it because of the use of prescription drugs? Did it happen because you were not familiar with portion control? Was it because you didn't have a good support system? Was it because you were constantly feeling stressed and overwhelmed? Was it because you did not have a proper structure or strategy in place?

We all have a story and until we look back, dig deeper and with the help of God know the source of our weight gain, then we will continue building on faulty foundation.

Losing weight is not just an outside job but an inside job too. I've stated before that weight gain could be linked to my childhood. I had grown up not feeling good enough, not feeling accepted (I was constantly compared to others, so I felt something was wrong with me), feeling rejected and feeling neglected. These feelings were at the root of my emotional eating. Junk food always gave me an escape route (a coping mechanism) and made me feel good when I was down, and that was how it all started. I had to go deeper and began with the help of God to work each problem out and renew my mind. Was it easy? No. Was it worth it?

Yes. Even up till now, I am constantly reminding myself of who I am in Christ and who I belong to. I no longer identify with being an emotional eater, I am a stable eater because I chose to address the root cause. Do I still get attacked by the devil in that area of my life every now and again? YES. The difference is that I now know what to do and just don't give him attention.

Give Up Your Excuses: I look back now, and I laugh at myself because I use to have a PHD in giving excuses and a master's degree in laziness. I would always find a reason why something couldn't be done. That reason would always make sense to me (who was I deceiving, of course me). If I couldn't proffer any reason, I would talk myself out of anything that was difficult. I hated the challenges in my life. The truth was that I just wanted things to be easy with no challenges. My excuses had to go because real life comes with challenges, and with the help of God I could and would overcome any that were thrown at me.

I began to see while on my journey that I usually made excuses because I was not asking God for wisdom to solve the problems I was facing; I would rely on my own strength which was never designed to take on life's challenges on its own. Once I began to ask God to help me each day, what looked like an excuse or obstacle became a steppingstone for me. Jesus said, "I am the way, the truth and life." Jesus – the way? It meant I could no longer be stranded. I always say it to myself "Seun there is always a way out or solution to every challenge if only you will look at it through the eyes of faith or your spiritual eyes."
The book of **James 1: 5 NIV,** says,

> *"If any of you lacks wisdom, you should ask God, who gives generously to all without finding fault, and it will be given to you."*

As I progressed on my journey, I would always tell myself that giving up was no longer an option, meaning no more excuses. It was painful in the beginning because I began to see that when I made those excuses, I was short-changing myself in growing, and failing to take responsibility for my life. I also began to see that the excuses were not really a stumbling block as they helped me think of better ways to solve some of the challenges I raised.

There are many reasons I made excuses and most of my excuses were rooted in the things listed below

- Fear of Failure/Making Mistakes – I did not want to start something, fail, and not complete it. If I made a mistake, then I'd be a failure.
- Fear of Embarrassment – The thought of being embarrassed if I did not attain what I was trying to do.
- Fear of Change – I hated change so much and losing weight meant I needed to be open to a totally new lifestyle.
- Fear of Uncertainty – I did not know what would happen, if I lost the weight would I be able to keep it off?
- Fear of Responsibility – I was always playing the blame game card. 'Well, I am an emotional eater because of the way I grew up.' This journey forced me to take ownership of my life.
- Perceived lack of confidence or resources – My confidence in my ability was zero plus being out of work at the beginning of the journey, I asked myself where the resources would come from.

Imagine the burden I willingly carried! The good news was that with God's help I overcame each one of them and I was able to renew my mind daily with His word.

Moses was one man that gave an excuse when God called him to lead the Israelites out of Egypt. His excuses centred on the fact that he couldn't speak, and God began to correct him immediately. Jeremiah also gave an excuse that he was too young when God called him. God immediately told him that He was sending him and that He would fortify him and make him strong on his journey. Gideon was another person who made an excuse when God called him to go and deliver the Israelites from the hands of the Midianites, he reminded God that he was the weakest in his family, but God refused to back down and showed him who he was by calling him a mighty warrior.

I found out that people in the Bible made excuses and it is natural for us as human beings to make excuses when things are way over our heads, but that is where God loves to come in and show Himself strong and mighty on our behalf. I have learnt that God will always call us for something way over our head so that we can rely on Him to do that which He is asking us to do. The only reason we make excuses is that we are looking at our own ability and not God's ability (supernatural ability).

During my journey God led me to a scripture that I memorised.
"I can do all things through Christ who strengthens me." (**Philippians 4: 13, NKJV**).

That scripture infused me with life, it made me see that I could lose weight through Christ who strengthens me and that was what killed my excuses. The excuses were valid, but with God's supernatural ability, I was able to overcome each one of them.

We often make excuses because we are focused on our natural strength and ability, but in Christ Jesus there is always a way out for us – children of God. We are children of God and we can tap into the ability and strength of Christ (the supernatural power within us) and do whatever our Father in heaven is asking us to do.

For example, I started writing this book during one of the difficult periods of my life, I had every excuse to just give up and not be bothered, but I knew God would give me the grace to write each day. I was committed and each day I showed up to write He was with me, which is what I call God's supernatural ability working in me. You need to bear in mind that I have never written a book before.

A few months after, I started work full time and I had another excuse not to write because I was always tired, and I just wanted to use the weekend to rest and prepare for the following week. I knew though, that if God called me to do something, He would give me the grace (supernatural strength) to do it. Once again, I asked Him to help me and He showed me how I could arrange my calendar to enable me write. I must confess though that on some days, I didn't feel like writing at all and some days I yearned to write. What I have learnt while writing this book is not to make excuses or follow my feelings, and to just keep pushing past the fear of never having written a book before.

We will always have an excuse not to do the right thing, but with the help of God we know that we can do all things through Christ who strengthens us.
Look at the areas in your life, situations where you would normally give excuses or talk yourself out of things, then ask God to help in those areas. God always give grace to the humble each time. Always remember you are a work-in-progress, don't beat yourself up when you make an excuse. Real victory is when you are now aware of those excuses you keep on making regarding your weight loss journey or lifestyle change, release them into God's hands and then ask Him to help you deal with them. Life will always present us an excuse each day and each moment, but we have the power in us to look at those excuses and turn them into opportunities. Excuses are opportunities in disguise!
Let me leave you with some quote on excuses.

"I attribute my success to this – I never gave up or took an excuse."
-Florence Nightingale

"Maturity is when you stop complaining and making excuses in your life; you

realize everything that happens in life is a result of the previous choice you've made and start making new choices to change your life." -**Roy T. Bennett**

"No one ever excused his way to success." -**Dave Del Dotto**

You have a Choice: Do you know that you have a choice? You can choose to be healthy or unhealthy. You can choose to eat your vegetables or not. You can choose to exercise your body or not. You can choose to be healed or not. You can choose to change your thought life or not. You have the ability to choose right in God. Life is governed by the decision to choose right daily. Always remember the secrets to your success are made by your daily choices. I have a choice to either write this book or not. If I didn't write it, it is still my choice but if I write it which I am doing now, it is still my choice and this choice will bless many people who will also choose to make up their mind to lose weight either now or in the future.

We often think that we don't have the power to make the right choice on our weight loss journey, so we give in easily by not doing what we know we ought to do, or we allow our feelings and emotions to overpower us. Frequently, we are led by our feelings rather than being led by the spirit (our inner being). When you become born again, your spirit is the one now in control not your flesh. God has given you the power to choose rightly each day and even when we make the wrong choices (which I did many times during my journey), He will gently correct us and pick us back up again. Always remember it is the little victories in the choices we make that become big wins. For instance, if you keep choosing to say no to all the wrong types of food being offered to you even though you have the right to eat them, it will eventually lead to big wins (weight loss). We usually don't know this, and we keep saying yes to all types of food offered to us without thinking, then we wonder why the weight is not shifting! This also applies to our emotions and our physical activities. Always remember the little 'no's always lead to the big wins.

Exercise Self-Control: I have talked about this in previous chapters and I must say this is one weapon you will need to use repeatedly. The truth is that as a Christian you can't use willpower to lose weight. It wouldn't work because you no longer live by your own strength and ability once you become born again. Your strength and ability cannot carry you far at all, even the Bible says, 'the human effort profits nothing but the words I speak to you are spirit and life.' (John 6: 63).

Self-control is a fruit of the spirit and you have it. Quite often, you might not even feel it because it can't be felt but it can only be activated by knowing God, He will reveal it to you. As a born-again Christian, you have the fruit of the spirit working in your spirit (inner being) daily, but for your soul and body to know this, it has to be revealed to you and you activate it through knowing. Once activated, as you use it daily you get stronger and stronger in it. The fruit of the spirit grows as you use it, so activate it and see how your weight loss journey will progress like never.

One Day at a Time: This became my motto! You can also adopt it and say it to yourself repeatedly. Losing weight and seeing results doesn't happen in a day or a month or a year or even years in some cases. People have underlying issues they are dealing with, but I know with God all things are possible. You will have to learn to be patient with yourself and be patient with the journey. I am yet to see anything that will last a long time being built quickly.

It took Noah between 80 – 100 years to build the ark, it took Solomon 20 years to build the temple and Jesus was 'built" (He lived) for 30 years in order to have a three-year ministry. It took Jesus three years to transform the disciples from being ordinary men into supernatural men. The best builder's work in this world is nothing compared to the way our God builds. When God builds, He is thinking of the many years to come and how your health will affect the next generations and how it will outlast you. Anything that involves God being the builder, designer, and creator, will take time because God always builds from the inside out and the best place to build is on Christ Jesus. When the storms of life come, they will really expose what your weight loss journey is built on. So please take it one day at a time with God. Whatever is worth building by God (including your weight loss journey) is worth building well one day at a time.

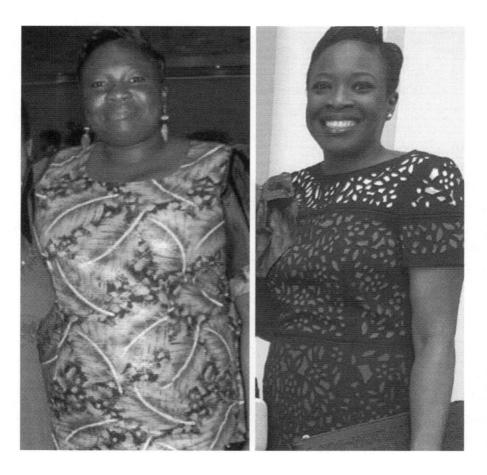

2009(Right),   2019(Left)

The Right Fuel, The Right Path And Staying The Course

Food is a gift from God, it is meant to energise and nourish our body. However only certain kinds of food truly nourish and are beneficial to our bodies. The Bible says in the book of **Genesis 2: 9, NIV**

"And the LORD God made all kinds of trees grow out of the ground – trees that were pleasing to the eye and good for food."

Eat Your Fruits and Vegetables: One habit you will have to cultivate is eating your fruits and vegetables. You can retrain your taste buds to love eating fruit and vegetables.

The NHS health message regarding the consumption of fruits and vegetables in the last 15 years has changed a lot. The NHS first recommended that everyone should have at least five portions of fruits and vegetables a day, but over the years new research from different sources have come out to say that we should be consuming seven to ten portions of fruits and vegetables a day. Who should we believe? My suggestion is for you to build up your fruits and vegetables intake one day at a time. There is no point trying to achieve seven portions of fruits and vegetables a day if you haven't even trained your taste buds to eat three to five portions a day. Start by getting vegetables into your main meals (lunch and dinner) and progress by ensuring you swap your snacks with fruits. As you do that, you are slowly retraining your appetite and before you know it your body will get use to eating fruits and vegetables.

The Balance Plate will help you when you use it at mealtimes to portion your ruits and vegetables, that way you know you are consuming enough. If you eat porridge for breakfast each morning, ensure you cut up a fruit (apple, banana, pear, grapes, pineapple) to sweeten it, that way you are also consuming a portion of your fruits and vegetables. Often, the reason why we don't love eating our fruits and vegetables is because we have fed our bodies with unhealthy food for so long and we have acquired a new taste. We can retrain our taste buds by eating the right food our body was created to eat. Even nature automatically tells us how good we feel whenever we feed our body the right food. You will feel better and lighter, your bowel movement will be frequent, your moods with be stable and you will also sleep better. The advantages are numerous. Your body was designed to consume fruit and vegetables, start giving it what it was designed to eat.

As stated above, eating fruits and vegetables provides many health benefits. People who eat more vegetables and fruits as part of an overall healthy diet are likely to have a reduced risk of some chronic diseases. Vegetables provide nutrients vital for health and maintenance of your body.

Why Consume Fruits and Vegetables?

- Fruits and vegetables are important sources of many nutrients our body needs daily to function well, including potassium, dietary fibre, folate (folic acid), vitamin A and vitamin C.
- Dietary fibre from vegetables, as part of an overall healthy diet, helps reduce blood cholesterol levels and may lower risk of heart disease. Fibre is important for proper bowel function. It helps reduce constipation. Fibre-containing foods such as vegetables help provide a feeling of fullness with fewer calories.
- As part of an overall healthy diet, eating foods such as vegetables that are lower in calories instead of some other higher-calorie food may be useful in helping to lower calorie intake.
- Eating food rich in vegetables and fruits as part of an overall healthy diet may

reduce risk for heart disease, including heart attack, stroke and may protect against certain types of cancers.

Colours of Fruits and Vegetables

You will get the most health benefits and protection against disease if you eat a wide variety of fruits and vegetables. The best way to eat your fruit and vegetables is to eat a wide range and rotate them weekly so that you can get different nutrients from them from time to time. Therefore, I will suggest you eat seasonal fruits and vegetables. The National Health Service in the UK introduced five-a-day portions of fruits and vegetables.

Foods of similar colours generally contain similar protective compounds. Try to eat a rainbow of colourful fruits and vegetables every day or weekly to get the full range of health benefits. For example:

- Red foods – like tomatoes and watermelon contain lycopene, which is thought to be important for fighting prostate cancer and heart disease.
- Green vegetables – like spinach and kale contain lutein and zeaxanthin which may help protect against age-related eye disease.
- Blue and purple foods – like blueberries and eggplant contain anthocyanins, which may help protect the body from cancer.
- White foods – like cauliflower contain sulforaphane and may also help protect against some cancers.

Selecting Fruits and Vegetables

To maximise nutrients and appeal, buy and serve different types of fruit and vegetables. Try to buy fruits and vegetables that are in season, choose fresh, frozen, or canned or tinned (choose the no added sugar and salt one). You should:

- Eat with the seasons – This is nature's way of making sure our bodies get a healthy mix of nutrients and vitamins we need.

Try something new – Try new recipes and buy new fruits or vegetables as part of your weekly shopping.

Let colours guide you – Get different combinations of nutrients by putting a 'rainbow' of colours (green, white, yellow, orange, purple, red etc) on your plate.

Looking for bargains – You can also shop at the farmers market to pick up your weekly essentials.

If you are struggling with your intake of fruits and vegetables don't give up, ask God to help open your eyes to see the reason behind it. You will be amazed what He will reveal to you. Try cooking your vegetables in different ways until you get to the one you like (steam, grill, pan fry etc). If you don't like eating whole fruits, look at cutting up your fruits into a small, lovely plate then eat it (this method works for lots of people). Don't give up and keep trying, you will end up loving fruits and vegetables. Your taste buds will not change overnight, so please give yourself lots of grace to change, remember it is a lifestyle change.

Put a Structure in Place: On my journey, I realised that I needed to have a structure in place that worked for me and that structure should also be subject to change when my season changed. When I started my journey of weight loss, I was working part time so I had a few days I could play with in terms of timing. Just a few months later I started a business and I needed to change my structure to accommodate the business timetable. Now I am working full time and I also have a business I am running at the side. I also have family, church, and volunteer responsibilities (I feel my hands are full, but I believe I have enough grace to carry it).

What do I mean by structure? Putting a structure in place means knowing what you should do with each day. Let me use myself as an example, after going back to full time employment, I realised that in order for my health to continuously be a priority, I needed to put a timetable in place or make a list for the day e.g., depending on the time I start work each day, I ensure I fit in about 30 minutes to 45 minutes of workout in the morning and take time out to take some short walks during the day or my lunch break. On my weekends I meal prep. I usually map out two to three hours on Saturday or Sunday night to meal prep. I will take time out on a Friday evening to write out a shopping list and draw up a food timetable. Most times, I follow the plan but sometimes I am happy to change to accommodate whatever is happening in my life at that moment. Consequently, I have staple foods (rice, beans, tinned fish, oats and pasta), frozen mixed veg and fruits in the freezer and I ensure I cook food in bulk for those days and store it in the freezer. Having this structure really helped me to know what I needed to do each day and not get distracted easily.

To write this book for example, I had to put a structure in place, I knew writing first thing in the morning or evening would not work for me, I took the opportunity to do most of my writing when I was transitioning from my old job into my new job. Since I started my new job, I had to put another structure in place to enable me write at the weekends or at times during my lunch breaks at work. I also used the Christmas period to write by taking some time off from work. I also began a 2-week holiday at the start of the COVID 19 pandemic, I took advantage of that time to write too.

I learnt also while writing this book that 'wishing' would not write it. I had to make it a priority and that was the only way I could get it done. If you need to wake up earlier please do, if you need to walk to work to get active, please do. If you need to get that personal trainer to motivate you, please do. If you need to be in an accountability group to inspire you, please do. Whatever you need to do, as the Lord lays it on your heart, do it, and ensure you prioritise your health and well-being. If you don't have a healthy body, you cannot fully carry out your God given assignment or purpose effectively.

Portion Control: Portion control is a concept that can be difficult to apply when you don't even know where to start from. Our food is now served in large portions whether we like it or not. The 'all you can eat' restaurants are not helping either, with the buffet table they lay out. The portions of most food supplied in the supermarkets have grown bigger and bigger over the years. Ask anyone who lived in the 30s, 40s or 50s, they will tell you how excessive our food portions have become as a nation over the years. Some of us grew up not knowing what portion control was – well I was one of them.

I am currently a Healthy Lifestyle Coach who facilitate several Health and Wellbeing programmes for the Borough of Barking and Dagenham. One important question that is often asked by people in all these programmes is what a portion should be like or what portion they can serve their children. You can see that portion control is a big problem as a nation. It is, however, a problem that can easily be solved.

There are several ways to control your portions which are counting calories, weighing the amount of food you eat, counting the macros in your food, using the measuring cup, or using different apps. The truth is they all work if you are consistent with them and you are ready to eat that way for the rest of your life. One of the several ways I usually advise or suggest is using the portion control or Balance Plate for both lunch time and dinner time. Half of your plate is vegetables or a salad, and the other half is split into two for carbs and protein. If you are new on your weight loss journey, apply this method (it works) and adjust your portions as you see fit for your physical activity level.

The reason why this way of eating works is because you are filling half of your plate with vegetables and salads which have extremely low calories, they are packed with nutrients and vitamins and they fill you up quicker. It also helps you to control your carb intake and protein intake (most of us struggle with our carbs and protein portions and eating this way will help you to control it). What is essential is the way we eat, which is portion control and what we eat – the type of food. These two go hand in hand, once we control our portions and we eat nutritionally dense food the weight will come off, our mood will lighten up and our emotions become stable.

Read Your Food Labels: Yes, I had to become a food label reader during my journey, and this continued even after it. This came about after I found the NHS website which enlightened me about what type of food needed to make it into my basket and what should not. I didn't know what to look out for in a product. If the packaging looked good or it said no added sugar or fat or just tasted nice, then it was good enough for me.

What I didn't know was that manufacturers were using sugar, salt, and fat to get me addicted to their products. Did you know that some pasta sauces have about seven teaspoons of sugar added to them? Did you know that most cereals in stores have more than five to six teaspoons of sugar added to them per 30g to 40g? Did you know that most crisps in stores are full of salt and unhealthy fats? Did you know that all food manufacturers are prohibited from giving false information when writing on the front of food packaging? When a food label says no added sugar, low in fat, helps you reduce your cholesterol, made with natural honey, high in fibre, high in protein, no added salt or oil, everything they have written in front on the food packaging is right and correct. What they do not tell you is that whenever they take something out, they always add something else to it. Once an item of food says low in fat on the packaging for example, what they have done is that they have replaced the fat with sugar. If you need to lose weight, you will have to become a food label reader and by doing this you will not be picking up the wrong food to buy. The purpose of you reading your food labels is to enable you to make the right food choices at any given time. Every food always has what they call a product label which usually gives you two sets of reliable information- the ingredients list and the nutrition informational panel – because we can trust the front of the packet messages.

Ingredients List – These are always ordered by weight so the first thing on this list is the main ingredients. For example, on a packet of bread the first ingredient is wholemeal flour or whole-wheat or whole grain, the second is water and third is yeast. This can help us to see how healthy a product is. If the first three or four are fat or sugar, you know the food is high in those ingredients, so it is a less healthy choice.

The Nutritional Information Panel – This is the table that gives you information about the energy (calories), protein, carbohydrate, and fat in food. It may also tell you the saturated fat, sugars, sodium, salt, and fibre content. The amounts are listed per 100g of food and sometimes per potions too.

Below is the UK food label government guideline to help you choose wisely. All food products that are on the green should go into your basket and always check that it is per 100g. When food packaging begins to show the orange and red sign below then you need to consider if it is really a healthy choice for you.

PUT A TRAFFIC LIGHT ON EVERY FOOD

All measures per 100g	LOW A healthier choice	MED OK most of the time	HIGH Just occasionally
Sugars	5g or less	5.1g – 22.5g	More than 22.5g
Fat	3g or less	3.1g – 17.5g	More than 17.5g
Saturates	1.5g or less	1.6g – 5g	More than 5g
Salt	0.3g or less	0.31g – 1.5g	More than 1.5g

High Fibre = 6g or more fibre per 100g

Another way that makes reading your food label easier for you is the Change4Life Food Scanner app which is downloadable for FREE from the iTunes store and Google Play.

The Change4Life food scanner works by scanning bar codes of food and drinks when you go shopping. Once an item has been scanned the app tells you how much sugar, salt and saturated fat is in the food you have scanned.

These include:

- Calorie information – The app tells you the number of calories in food and drink products and will also provide calorie information per serving suggestion.
- Improved results layout – You will find it much easier to understand what's in your food after scanning.

The Change4Life food scanner made it so much easier for me. Once the food is scanned, it tells me if it is a yes or no immediately. Reading your food labels will help you make wise choices that will enhance your weight loss journey. Do you want to lose weight and know you are making the right food choices? Then start reading your labels and half of your weight loss or health problems are already solved?

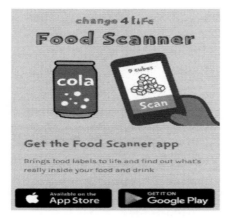

Be Sugar Smart: What exactly is sugar? It can be confusing – we use the word to talk about the sugar in our food, the sugar we add to our foods, carbohydrates, and our blood sugar level. It is all these things. The simple form of sugar (glucose) is the main fuel for our body. Glucose is released into our bloodstream (as blood sugar or blood glucose) when we digest starchy foods and circulates around the body to give us energy. Since sugar is produced when we digest starchy foods and is naturally in fruits and dairy products, we don't need to consume many foods and drinks containing added sugar. In the same way, we don't need to add extra sugar ourselves. On my journey I had to become the sugar police. I have mentioned this before in previous chapters, I used to drink up to three 500ml bottles of coke a day. In addition to that I would drink a 500ml bottle of Lucozade drink or a hot chocolate drink. I ate cakes, biscuits and other sauces that accompanied my £1.99 chicken and chips. I was an added sugar addict because all the food I loved contained added sugar, from fizzy drinks to biscuits to cakes to sauces to hot drinks. At the start of my weight loss journey, I didn't realise that I could retrain my taste buds to stop being addicted to added sugar. One of the ways I achieved that was becoming sugar smart.

Did you know that regularly consuming foods and drinks high in sugar increases your risk of obesity and tooth decay? In a study published in 2014 in JAMA Internal Medicine, Dr Hu and his colleagues found an association between a high-sugar diet and a greater risk of dying from heart disease. Over the course of the 15-year study, people who got 17% to 21% of their calories from added sugar had a 38% higher risk of dying from cardiovascular disease compared with those who consumed 8% of their calories as added sugar.
"Basically, the higher the intake of added sugar, the higher the risk for heart disease," says Dr Hu.

Consuming too much added sugar can raise blood pressure and increase chronic inflammation, both of which are pathological pathways to heart disease. Excess consumption of sugar, especially in sugary beverages, also contributes to weight gain by tricking your body into turning off its appetite-control system because liquid calories are not as satisfying as calories from solid foods. Therefore, it is easier for people to add more calories to their regular diet when consuming sugary beverages.

"The effects of added sugar intake - higher blood pressure, chronic inflammation, obesity and metabolic syndrome, high cholesterol, Type 2 diabetes, and fatty liver disease, dental plaque and cavities - are all linked to an increased risk for heart attack and stroke," says Dr Hu. Excessive sugar consumption has links to several harmful health conditions.

Currently, children and adults across the UK are consuming more than a healthy amount of sugar. However, if there is too much sugar in your meals, you are also less likely to get all the nutrients you need. That is because added sugar contains empty calories – energy without much or no nutrition. This also means that sugary food often doesn't fill you up, so you have consumed lots of calories but might still want to eat more. Which will fill you more quickly? A bar of chocolate or slice of cake or an apple? Of course, we all know it is an apple that will fill us more because of the fibre in it. Sugary food isn't as filling as nutrient rich foods, so they can cause you to eat more calories than you realise or need for your body. Use the food label to help you choose foods lower in sugar.

What are the differences between natural sugar and added sugar?

There are different names for sugar, and they can be divided into natural sugar (these are naturally found in our fruits and dairy products) and added sugar (these are added to food to make them sweeter e.g. cakes, biscuits, and sauces – they contain added sugar which come in different names).

Natural Sugar

Fruit sugar – (fructose) fresh fruits, tinned fruits, dried fruits, fresh fruits juice, fresh homemade smoothies; milk sugar (lactose) milk, yoghurts, cheese, and other dairy products.

Fact – fruits are full of important vitamins, minerals, and fibre, so include them in your diet in healthy portions. Dairy products are important for our bones.

Added Sugar

Glucose – used in many sweet foods and drinks, especially ones that use a liquid form of sugar such as boiled sweets, cakes, and energy drinks.

Sucrose – used in hot drinks, sweets, cakes, biscuits, jams, marmalades, sweet spread, sweet bread, sweet pastries (croissants and danish pastries), ice cream, sauces (ketchups, brown sauce, sweet chilli sauce), desserts, puddings, and other baked goods.

Non-alcoholic drink – Fizzy drinks, fruits squashes, high juices, fruit juices (concentrated), sweetened drinks like milkshakes, yoghurts drinks and alcoholic drinks.

Fact – There is no nutritional reason to have high glucose food and drinks and it is also unhealthy to have too much of it in your food.

Different names for added sugar are listed below.

Sucrose, Glucose, Lactose, Fructose, Dextrose, Maltose, Glucose, Fructose syrup, Molasses, Honey, Golden syrup, Maple syrup, Corn Syrup, Sugar Syrup, Treacle, Agave etc.

What has happened over the years is that food manufacturers have used different names to disguise sugar. Just because a product doesn't list sugar as one of the ingredients in it doesn't mean it doesn't have any. Watch out for the alternative names for sugar mentioned above in the ingredient listing on the pack of each food item you purchase. You can be sugar smart.

Tips For Reducing Sugar Intake

- Take it slow by reducing your added sugar intake gradually. It may help to start by eliminating the most obvious sources of sugar. You can easily avoid baked goods such as cakes, muffins, and brownies. Removing sweets, chocolate and sugary beverages is also an excellent place to start.

- Swap sugary cereals (e.g. granola, cluster, and chocolate cereals) with no added sugar muesli, plain porridge, or homemade granola.

- Replace added sugar with sweet tasting herbs and spices, common replacements include cinnamon, nutmeg, cardamom, and vanilla. These can be a flavoursome addition to coffee, oatmeal, or yogurt.

- Look at the ingredients list, if sugar is in the top three to four list ingredients, do not buy it.

- If you fancy something sweet to eat, choose low sugar options e.g. fruits, homemade ice cream made with yogurts and topped with fruits.

- Check whether a product is low in sugar using the label reader of the Change4life app before buying it.

- Don't buy food high in sugar and don't add sugar to your food.

- Replacing fizzy drinks, flavoured water, concentrated fruit juice, hot chocolate with unsweetened herbal tea, coffee without sugar, sparkling mineral water, or just water.

- Avoid adding sugary savoury sauces (e.g. tomato and brown sauces, sweet chili sauce and herbs and spice mixes with added sugar)

- Instead of adding sugar in recipes, use extracts like cinnamon, vanilla, orange, or lemon.

- Instead of adding sugar to cereal or oatmeal, try fresh fruit (e.g. bananas, cherries, or strawberries) or dried fruit (raisins, cranberries or apricots).

- Switch out sugar with unsweetened applesauce, dates in recipes (use equal amounts).

- Focus on eating whole foods like vegetables, fruits, whole, unprocessed grains and legumes, lean protein and nuts and seeds.

Do you know that 4g of sugar is equal to one teaspoon of sugar? The table below tells us the amount of added sugar that is secretly added to the drinks we consume daily. Be sugar smart, the weight will fall off and your health will improve greatly.

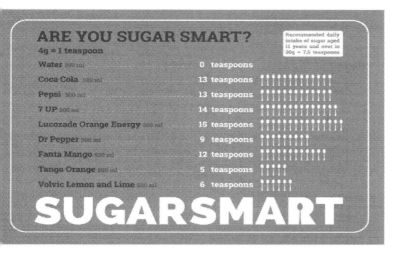

Picture and content owned by Sugar Smart

Swap Unhealthy Food With Healthy Food: The food industry is full of unhealthy food which will not aid your weight loss journey. The good news is that you can swap unhealthy food with healthy food, and you will lose weight and become healthy. One thing I had to do on my journey was to immediately swap my fizzy drinks with water and it has been one of the best decisions I have ever made.

No one is saying you can't eat the same things you have been eating, all that I am advising is to look for a healthy alternative or you create a healthy alternative. Let's say for example you love Chinese food (chicken chow mein), do you know you can recreate yours and make it even healthier? At least you can control what is going into the meal. I love chicken and chips, and it was very easy for me to pick it up on my way home for £1.99. Now I have chosen consistently to make it each time I feel like eating it and that decision has really aided my weight loss. Your taste buds will not automatically love the swap but if you persevere for a while, they will start to love it.

With the sugar smart campaign spreading all over the UK now, food manufacturers are now willing to offer healthy alternatives to consumers, and we can also see the emergence of new companies that are now offering healthier drinks, snacks and food. Let's consider breakfast cereals for example, an average breakfast cereal of 30g to 40g has about six teaspoons of sugar in it, but guess what? You can swap sugary breakfast cereals for plain cereals such as plain porridge, shredded whole wheat, homemade granola (I make mine and they come out perfectly) or no added sugar muesli. Swap flavoured or corner-style yoghurts for plain yoghurts and sweeten them by adding fresh fruit inside. You can swap your white rice, pasta, bread for brown or wholegrain rice, pasta, or bread.

I have put the table blow to help you see the different ways that you can swap your snacks or desserts or drinks.

Snacks Or Dessert

Swap this	For this
Flavoured chips or crackers	Veggie sticks (Carrot, red pepper etc) and dip like hummus, avocado mash, kale chips, homemade plantain chips, homemade popcorn
Biscuit/Cookie	Sliced pear or apple with 100% nut butter or homemade biscuits
Pudding or custard	Chia seed pudding
Ice cream	Plain dairy or coconut yoghurt with berries, or a small serve of homemade smoothie bowl (use frozen banana as the base – it's good!)
Cake, slice or chocolate bar	Fruits, hardboiled egg, nuts etc
Snack bar, muesli bar or fruit snacks	Pick 'n' mix of your favourite raw nuts, seeds and other yummy bits like coconut chips and a little dried fruit

Drinks

Swap this	For this
Flavoured chips or crackers	Plain water or water infused with fruit pieces and fresh herbs
Biscuit/Cookie	Plain semi skimmed or skimmed milk, oat milk, almond, or hazelnut milk all unsweetened
Juice	Water infused with fruit pieces and fresh herbs
Flavoured coffee, hot chocolate, sugary tea	Black coffee, or plain coffee, fruit or herbal tea, 100% cocoa drink with no added sugar

Lower Your Salt Intake: Eating too much salt has been linked to high blood pressure, which causes damage to your blood vessels and arteries when chronically elevated. In turn, this increases your risk of heart disease, stroke, heart failure and kidney disease. Even if you rarely put salt on your meals, you could be getting too much salt just from your food. In fact, 75% of the salt we eat is already in our food (this is often the same food that is full of unhealthy fat). To keep your heart healthy, it's important that you don't eat too much salt each day.

How much is too much?

Adults should eat less than six grams of salt each day, that's about one teaspoon. This includes the salt that's contained within readymade foods like bread, as well as the salt you add during cooking and at the table.

How do I know how much salt I'm eating?

One of the best ways to work out how much salt you're eating is to check the food label or nutritional information on the packaging of any food you're buying or eating. If you're buying any food, look at the 'amount per serving' to see how much salt is in the food.

How much is too much per 100g?

	Low	Medium	High
Salt	0g - 0.3g	0.3g - 1.5g	More than 1.5g
Sodium	0g - 0.1g	0.1g - 0.6g	More than 0.6g

Food doesn't need to be tasteless or bland. There are lots of things you can do to make sure your food is still exciting and satisfying.

- Check the nutritional information on food labels and try to pick low-salt options and ingredients.
- Add less salt when cooking and don't add salt to your food at the table. As you get used to the taste of food without salt, cut it out completely.
- Flavour your food with pepper, fresh herbs, garlic, ginger, spices, or lemon juice instead.
- Taste your food first, it may not need salt.
- Watch out for cooking sauces and seasonings like soy sauce or jerk seasoning – some of these are very high in salt.
- Swap salty snacks such as crisps and salted nuts with fruit, vegetables, or raw nuts instead.
- Avoid saltier foods such as bacon, cheese, takeaways, ready meals, and other processed food.

Reduce Your Fat Intake: In the last few years, fat has been given a bad name or reputation. When we hear the word fat, what comes to our mind automatically is the word 'bad'. Fat is not bad, what may be bad is the type of fat we eat, which means we need to re-educate ourselves about different types of fat, which one is good for us and what quantity of it we need to eat. We need a number of fatty acids and fat soluble (e.g. vitamins A, D, E) are essential for our bodies – normally for our cells, hormones, eyes, brain, and skin; and it should be eaten as part of a healthy lifestyle. However, we can see from the Eatwell Plate guide in chapter nine, that oils and fats should make up the smallest part of our eating portion.

It's important to for me to emphasise at this stage that certain types of fat are good for you – they are healthy. I was a novice when it came to what type of fats were good for the body or not, what the role of fat was and what quantity the body needs. The old me, would just pour oil into my food without thinking (I am sure many Africans can relate to this). Most of the food I cooked was fried, and I always bought fried food on the go. On my journey to a healthier me, I had to re-educate myself about the quantity I needed to consume, what type of fat I needed to eat and why most of my fat needed to come from food.

Fat is a major source of energy and supports balanced hormones. A small amount of fat is an essential part of a healthy, balanced diet. Fat is a source of essential fatty acids, which the body cannot make itself. Fat helps the body absorb vitamin A, vitamin D and vitamin E. These vitamins are fat-soluble, meaning they can only be absorbed with the help of fats. Any fat not used by your body's cells or to create energy is converted into body fat. All types of fat are high in energy. A gram of fat, whether saturated or unsaturated, provides 9kcal (37kJ) of energy compared with 4kcal (17kJ) for carbohydrates and protein.

The main types of fat found in food are:

- Saturated fats - Saturated Fats & Trans fats
- Unsaturated fats – Monounsaturated & Polyunsaturated

Most fats and oils contain both saturated and unsaturated fats in different proportions. As part of a healthy diet, we should cut down on foods and drinks high in saturated fats and trans fats and replace them with unsaturated fats.

Saturated Fats

Saturated fats are found in many foods both sweet and savoury. Most of them come from animal sources including meat, and dairy products, and are usually solid at room temperature as well as some plants foods, coconut oil.

Foods high in saturated fats include.

- Fatty cuts of meat
- Meat products, including sausages and pies
- Chicken skin or crackling
- Full cream dairy products including butter, ghee and lard
- Cream, soured cream and ice cream
- Some savoury snacks, like cheese crackers and some popcorns
- Chocolate confectionery
- Biscuits, cakes, and pastries
- Coconut oil, cream, or milk

Trans Fats

These occur naturally in some foods but are also formed when vegetables oils go through a process called hydrogenation – when liquid oils are turned into solid fats. This is used in food production to increase the shelf life of processed products (e.g. making a cake last for weeks instead of days). Trans fats are considered bad for our health because they increase the amount of LDL (low-density lipoprotein or bad cholesterol) and decrease the amount of HDL (high-density lipoprotein or good cholesterol) therefore increasing our risk of heart disease.

Unsaturated Fats

If you want to cut your risk of heart disease, it's best to reduce your overall fat intake and swap saturated fats for unsaturated fats. There's good evidence that suggests replacing saturated fats with some unsaturated fats can help lower cholesterol.

ound primarily in oils from plants and fish, unsaturated fats can be either polyunsaturated or monounsaturated.

Monounsaturated Fat: It help protect our hearts by maintaining levels of good cholesterol while reducing levels of bad cholesterol.
Monounsaturated fats are found in:

Olive oil, rapeseed oil, sesame oil, peanut oil, and canola oil

Avocados

Nuts such as almonds nuts, brazils nuts, peanuts, and seeds etc.

Polyunsaturated Fats: It can help lower the level of LDL cholesterol, these fats come from vegetables, plants and fish and are also often in liquid form at room temperature. Some polyunsaturated fats are essential for health and cannot be made by the body, so we must eat them to have a healthy diet.

There are two main types of polyunsaturated fats: Omega-3 and Omega-6.
Some types of Omega-3 and Omega-6 fats cannot be made by the body and are therefore essential in small amounts in the diet.
Omega-6 fats are found in vegetable oils, such as:

Rapeseed

Sunflower

Some nuts

Omega-3 fats are found in oily fish, such as:

Kippers

Herring

Trout

Sardines

Salmon

Mackerel

- Pilchards
- Fresh Tuna

They are also found in walnuts, seeds, soya beans, green leafy vegetables, and linseed.

Most of us get enough omega-6 in our diet, but we're advised to have more omega-3 by eating at least two portions of fish a week, including one portion of oily fish.

Omega-3 fats are a type of polyunsaturated fat that, like other dietary polyunsaturated fats, can help to reduce your risk of heart disease. Omega-3 fats can:
- Lower heart rate and improve heart rhythm
- Decrease the risk of clotting
- Lower triglycerides
- Reduce blood pressure
- Improve blood vessel function and delay the build-up of plaque (a fatty substance) in coronary arteries.

Cut Back on Fat: We consume fat in all sorts of ways. Some people eat more crisps and chocolate, whereas others use a lot of oil in cooking, others eat more fatty meats or choose creamy salad dressings. We have identified three main ways that fat comes into our diet.
- Eating foods with inbuilt fat (e.g. meat or chocolate bars)
- The way we cook our food (e.g. frying)
- Adding fat food when cooking (e.g. butter and vegetables)

When choosing or preparing high fats foods:
- Ask at the counter or market for leaner cuts of meats, take the skin off poultry

and remove all visible fat before cooking.

- Eat fewer crisps and other high fats snacks food (e.g. salted peanuts, chips, takeaway, pastries, and chocolate)
- Choose low fat dairy products, skimmed milk, reduced fat cheese or plant base etc.
- Plan swaps – choose a side salad instead of onion rings with your burger.
- When cooking:
- Grill, bake, roast, steam or poach instead of frying food.
- Avoid deep frying and deep-fried foods.
- Invest in a non-stick pan or wok – you will require much less oil.
- Just because a recipe asks for fats or oil, it doesn't mean you can't use less or swap it for a lower fat variety (one teaspoon of cooking oil can have over 40 calories, but spray oil contains just one calorie per spray)

Before adding extra fats:

- Measure out fat added to foods using a teaspoon or switch to a spray oil.
- Use balsamic vinegar, oil free dressing or a drizzle of lemon or lime juice to dress salads and meals. This gives plenty of flavour without excess fat and calories.
- Check food labels to make sure the dressings, oils, and butter you choose are low fat.
- Choose pickles, chutneys etc as they are often lower in fat than rich sauces, gravies, and salad dressings.

Drink up to six to eight Glasses of Water a Day: Your body needs water or other fluids to work properly and to avoid dehydration. About 60% of your body weight is made of water. You need it for every single bodily function. It flushes toxins from your organs, carries nutrients to your cells, cushions your joints, and helps you digest the food you eat. That's why it's important to drink enough fluids. In climates such as the UK's, we should drink about 1.2 litres (six to eight glasses) of fluid every day to stop us getting dehydrated according to the NHS. In hotter climates, the body needs more than this. I struggled with drinking water, but I didn't give up and I asked the Lord to help when I made up my mind to lose weight.

Our body has been designed to love water and the reason a lot of us struggle with this is because over the years, we have reconditioned our taste buds to love sugary drinks. The truth is that the body will thank you when you make up your mind to drink water and with God's help, and prayers (prayers work wonders) you will change.

Did you know that you have to try a new food or drink 10 – 12 times before your taste buds can decide whether they really like the food or not? That means that you have to try a new food 10 – 12 times before you can say you don't like it. It must be ten different times – not ten bites at the same meal! So, you see you can learn to love to drink water. Start by drinking cool water and if you don't like it, change to warm water and if you don't like it add lemon to it, and if you still don't like it infuse it with fruit. Your body was designed by God to drink water and not consume sugary drinks. Give your body the best it deserves and see how it will begin to function well.

Everyone's needs are unique to them and depend on their health, age, size, and weight as well as activity levels, the type of job they do and the climate they live in. Drinking a little but often is the best way to stay hydrated. In the UK, the Eatwell Guide suggests you should aim for 6-8 glasses of water and other liquids each day to replace normal water loss around 1.2 to 1.5 litres. Water, sugar-free drinks, including tea and coffee all count.

In March 2010, the **European Food Safety Authority (EFSA)** issued a report suggesting an adequate total daily intake of two litres of fluids for women and 2.5

itres for men. This quantity includes drinking water, drinks of all kinds and the moisture available from the food we eat. On average our food is thought to contribute about 20% of our fluid intake which, therefore, suggests a woman should aim to drink about 1.6 litres and a man should aim for two litres.

However, there is controversy surrounding our hydration needs. Some argue that there's a lack of scientific evidence to support the perceived health benefits of drinking the often-touted two litres a day, especially when it comes to those of us who live in temperate climates and who lead a largely sedentary lifestyle. However, the NHS still recommends that we consume around 6-8 glasses, with more required in hot weather or if exercising.

Do Liquids Other than Water Count?

Water, milk, sugar-free drinks and tea and coffee all count but remember that caffeinated drinks like tea and coffee can make the body produce urine more quickly. Fruit juice and smoothies also count but because they contain 'free' sugars (the type we are encouraged to cut back on), you should limit these to a combined total of 150ml per day. Many of the foods we eat contribute to our fluid intake – for example, dishes like soup as well as fruit and vegetables with a high-water content, such as melons, courgettes or cucumbers.

Health Benefits of Drinking Enough Water

- Weight loss: Drinking enough water may help you burn more calories, reducing appetite if consumed before a meal and lowering the risk of long-term weight gain.
- Better physical performance: Modest dehydration may impair physical performance. Losing only 2% of your body's water content during exercise may increase fatigue and reduce motivation.
- Reduced severity of headaches: For those prone to headaches, drinking additional water may reduce the intensity and duration of episodes. In

dehydrated individuals, water may help relieve headache symptoms.

- Constipation relief and prevention: In people who are dehydrated, drinking enough water may help prevent and relieve constipation.
- Decreased risk of kidney stones: Although more research is needed, there is some evidence that increasing water consumption may help prevent recurrence in people with a tendency to form kidney stones.
- Gets rid of wastes through urination, perspiration, and bowel movements: Research shows that drinking water help to flush out toxins in the body daily.

Tips –Do you know that drinking water about a half hour before meals can also reduce the number of calories you end up consuming? Now that you know you can try it, it works. One study showed that people who were looking to lose weight who drank one glass of water before each meal lost 44% more weight over 12 weeks, compared to those who didn't. Overall, it seems that drinking adequate amounts of water, particularly before meals, may have a benefit.

Try it, I know it works, it is tips like this that makes your weight loss journey easier. Refuse to buy into the lie that you don't like water, your body was designed to live on water. Choose today to train your taste buds to start loving water. Always remember Rome was not built in a day.

Plan of Action

By now you will have started seeing changes once you've started working on your goals in Book One. Book Two is structured to guide and equip you on your weight loss journey or living a healthier/balanced lifestyle.

1. **What are the three most important areas that you really want to see a change? E.g. making good choices, learning how to overcome temptation, trusting God for supernatural provision etc.**

   a. _____

   b. _____

   c. _____

2. **State below which one of the three is your top priority.**

   I commit to working on..

   ....

   Remember you are making a commitment to yourself.

3. What plan have you put in place to achieve this goal?

4. What are the challenges or pitfalls that may stop you from achieving this goal?

5. What are the solutions you could use to overcome these challenges?

6. What support system do you have in place – friends, family, accountability *group, colleagues at work?*

7. I will review this goal on

....

Once you have achieved the first goal on your list, go and pick another one out of the top three and begin to work on it.

"*It does not matter how slowly you go as long as you do not stop.* "– **Confucius**

Even the snail entered Noah's ark, so keep going. Always remember with Christ you can do all things through Him who strengthens you.

Book
Three

Exercise/Physical Activity-the Miracle Cure

Getting physically active is a human necessity, being physically active is a need for the body and not a want. Exercise is the miracle cure we've always had, but for too long we've neglected to take our recommended dose. Our health is now suffering as a consequence. Whatever your age, there's strong scientific evidence that being physically active can help you lead a healthier and happier life.

People who exercise regularly have a lower risk of developing many long-term (chronic) conditions, such as heart disease, Type 2 diabetes, stroke, and some cancers. It can reduce your risk of major illnesses such as heart disease, stroke, Type 2 diabetes and cancer by up to 50% and lower your risk of early death by up to 30%.

Research shows that physical activity can also boost self-esteem, mood, sleep quality and energy, as well as reducing your risk of stress, depression, dementia and Alzheimer's disease. In fact, a study in 24 women who had been diagnosed with depression showed that exercise of any intensity significantly decreased feelings of depression. The effects of exercise on mood are so powerful that choosing to exercise (or not) even makes a difference over short periods.

One study asked 26 healthy men and women who normally exercised regularly to either continue exercising or stop exercising for two weeks. Those who stopped exercising experienced increases in negative mood "If exercise were a pill, it would be one of the most cost-effective drugs ever invented," says Dr Nick Cavill, a health promotion consultant.

Our body has been designed by God to have movement each day, not each week or month or year. **1 Timothy 4: 8, NLT** says,

"Physical training is good, but training for godliness is much better, promising benefits in this life and in the life to come."

The **Merriam-Webster** dictionary defines the word *'good'* as pleasant advantageous, wholesome, profitable, suitable, fit, honourable, right, and commendable. God Himself has endorsed physical training as **good.** We live in a world that leaves us no time to get physically active. Our life is so busy that getting physically active is the least on our mind, yet God who formed us, created us in His own image is telling us that being physically active is a good thing. Yet, we allow the world to tell us how to live and not conform to the way God has designed us to live. Now is the time to make up your mind to be physically active and trust me, when God says something is good, there is no point arguing just obey and ask Him to give you the grace to do what He has asked you to do.

People are less active nowadays, partly because technology has made our lives easier. We drive cars or take public transport. Machines wash our clothes. We entertain ourselves in front of a TV or computer screen. Fewer people are doing manual work, and most of us have jobs that involve little physical effort. Work, household chores, shopping and other necessary activities are far less demanding than for previous generations. We move around less and burn off less energy than people use to.

Research suggests that many adults spend more than seven hours a day sitting down, at work, on transport or in their leisure time. People aged over 65 spend ten hours or more each day sitting or lying down, making them the most sedentary age group. Inactivity is described by the Department of Health as a "silent killer". Evidence is emerging that sedentary behaviour, such as sitting or lying down for long periods, is bad for your health. Not only should you try to raise your activity levels, but you should also reduce the amount of time you and your family spend sitting down. Common examples of sedentary behaviour include watching TV, using a computer, using the car for short journeys, and sitting down to read, talk or listen to music. This type of behaviour is thought to increase your risk of developing many chronic diseases, such as heart disease, stroke and Type 2 diabetes, as well as weight gain and obesity. "Previous generations were active more naturally through work and manual labour, but today we have to find ways of integrating activity into our daily lives," says Dr Cavill. Whether it's limiting the time babies spend strapped in their buggies, or encouraging adults to stand up and move frequently, people of all ages need to reduce their sedentary behaviour. "This means that each of us needs to think about increasing the types of activities that suit our lifestyle and can easily be included in our day," says Dr Cavill.

I was never physically active. My job at that time involved me sitting most of the time and it was easy to take some means of transportation from one place to another. The phrase physically active was strange to me. I decided to start exercising at home even though I gave up few times. My friend Bayo told me it was okay to feel that way, but I had to always finish what I started. I had to be patient with myself. I didn't even have the right workout gear (I would wear an old t-shirt, shorts, and old trainers) but I still chose to give it a go. After trying it quite a few times, I began to reap the benefits of being physically active and that is still what motivates me to exercise till today. I often don't feel like it, but I have learnt over the years not to yield to my feelings. Instead I do what is right which is getting physically active, and always remember you only get the reward after your obedience. You can retrain your feelings to do the right thing at all times, it might start off hard but with the help of God it will get easier. God knows it will be hard for you and that is why He has given you the Holy Spirit to strengthen and equip you.

Always remember motivation gets you started, but it is habit and discipline that keep you going. Stop replying on motivation all the time. I am never motivated to do 90% of the things I do now, I do them because it is the right thing to do. You can ask God to help you on this journey and He will make it easier every step of the way as you rely on Him.

It's important for us to know the benefits of being physically active. I have come to understand with my body that what I sow is what I reap. If I choose to sow being physically active over a long period of time, I will reap good health and a number of the things listed below.

Benefits of Regular Physical Activity

Given the overwhelming evidence, it seems obvious that we should all be physically active. It's essential if you want to live a healthy and fulfilling life into old age.

It's medically proven that people who do regular physical activity enjoy the following:

- Up to a 35% lower risk of coronary heart disease and stroke
- Up to a 50% lower risk of Type 2 diabetes
- Up to a 50% lower risk of colon cancer
- Up to a 20% lower risk of breast cancer
- A 30% lower risk of early death
- Up to an 83% lower risk of osteoarthritis
- Up to a 68% lower risk of hip fracture
- A 30% lower risk of falls (among older adults)
- Up to a 30% lower risk of depression
- Help you to control weight
- Improves your mood
- Exercise boosts your energy
- Promotes better sleep

- Exercise puts the spark back into your sex life
- Increases mental health and social well being
- Live longer—up to five years according to the **American Journal of Preventative Medicine!**

Moderate or strong evidence for health benefit

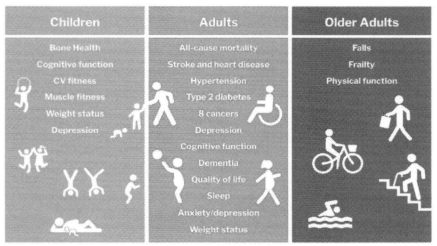

Children	Adults	Older Adults
Bone Health	All-cause mortality	Falls
Cognitive function	Stroke and heart disease	Frailty
CV fitness	Hypertension	Physical function
Muscle fitness	Type 2 diabetes	
Weight status	8 cancers	
Depression	Depression	
	Cognitive function	
	Dementia	
	Quality of life	
	Sleep	
	Anxiety/depression	
	Weight status	

Now that we have spoken about why we need to be physically active and the benefits, I am sure you will be wondering what type of physical activity you can do. There are lots of things you can do.

In September 2019, the UK Chief Medical Officer released an updated report of physical activity guidelines in the UK for all age groups from children to adult, to pregnant women to physically challenged people to older women. The report is a guideline to help us become more active as a nation and the reasons why it is urgent for us now.

According to this report, which was released in 2019, to stay healthy, adults should try to be active every day and aim to achieve at least 150 minutes of physical activity over a week through a variety of activities. If broken down, it is about 30 min a day. For most people, the easiest way to get moving is to make activity part of everyday life, like walking or cycling instead of using the car to get around. However, the more you do, the better; and taking part in activities such as sports and exercise will make you even healthier.

For any type of activity to benefit your health, you need to be moving quick enough to raise your heart rate, breathe faster and feel warmer. This level of effort is called **moderate intensity activity.** If you're working out at a moderate intensity you should still be able to talk, but you won't be able to sing the words to a song.

An activity where you have to work even harder is called **vigorous intensity activity.** There is substantial evidence that vigorous activity can bring health benefits over and above that of moderate activity. You can tell when it's vigorous activity because you're breathing hard and fast, and your heart rate has gone up quite a bit. If you are working out at this level, you won't be able to say more than a few words without pausing for a breath.

The examples given below are provided as a guide only and will vary between individuals.

Moderate Activities (I can talk while I do them, but I can't sing.)	Vigorous Activities (I can only say a few words without stopping to catch my breath.)
• Ballroom and line dancing • Biking on level ground or with few hills • Canoeing • General gardening (raking, trimming shrubs) • Sports where you catch and throw (baseball, softball, volleyball) • Tennis (doubles) • Using your manual wheelchair • Using hand cyclers—also called ergometers • Walking briskly • Water aerobics	• Aerobic dance • Biking faster than 10 miles per hour • Fast dancing • Heavy gardening (digging, hoeing) • Hiking uphill • Jumping rope • Martial arts (such as karate) • Race walking, jogging, or running • Sports with a lot of running (basketball, hockey, soccer) • Swimming fast or swimming laps • Tennis (singles)

I'm sure at this stage you'll probably be wondering, what type of physical exercise you should do. It's advisable to start with taking a long walk each morning. You can even turn it to prayer walking – walking at the same time speaking to God and also learning how to quiet your mind. Later, you can try something else until you find what suits your current lifestyle.

I have come across people who didn't set a foot in the gym but have lost weight just by choosing to do some brisk walking. I coached a lady few years ago, who lost weight just by ensuring she did over 6,000 steps a day while also eating healthy. She lost over 10kg within six months! Always remember one size does not fit all. If I use myself as an example, 90% of time I work out at home. What I do is create a 60 to – 90-day challenge for myself, I'll go on YouTube and look for the type of physical activity I would love to challenge my body with then put a plan in place. Always remember psychical activity doesn't happen until you plan it, take some time out the night before or on a Sunday and plan your workout as you would plan when meal prepping. Put it on your to-do list for the week and once you have done it, tick it off your list. You will have a sense of accomplishment one you have completed your workout.

You can also start by taking a long walk for about 30 minutes to one hour each day, if you need to wake up early then do it. If you try walking and it is not for you, try buying/downloading an exercise app on your phone or search YouTube, it has over 100,000 worth of free exercise videos. One thing I will advise is that you keep trying new things until you find the workout that suits your current lifestyle. If none of the suggestions above work then join a gym, get a personal trainer to show you how to use the equipment, try swimming (most gyms have swimming sessions), try water aerobics, try dancing, sign up for a 5k or 10k (a half marathon or full marathon) to keep you challenged as your gain more strength. You can also try finding a running buddy or joining a running club. Once you find what works for you, stick with it, be patient and consistent; you will see the weight come off and it becomes a lifestyle. Keep taking one day at a time until you find what works for you. Always remember quitting is not an option.

The Bottom Line

- Exercise offers incredible benefits that can improve nearly every aspect of your health from the inside out.
- Regular physical activity can increase the production of hormones that make you feel happier and help you sleep better.
- It can also improve your skin's appearance, help you lose weight and keep it off, lessen the risk of chronic disease and improve your sex life.
- Whether you practice a specific sport or follow the guideline of 150 minutes of activity per week, you will inevitably improve your health in many ways.

The Way To A Better You

In becoming a healthier and a better you, one of the things you must learn to embrace is change. This may be hard, but it is necessary on your weight loss journey.

We have discussed earlier about embracing change through our habits. It will feel hard at the beginning of your weight loss journey to develop a new habit and trust me I can relate to this. One thing I will advise is that you should never decide to change all your habits at once, otherwise you will feel overwhelmed and immediately give up. You need to understand that changing your habits require a lot of mental strength and commitment. It is easy to exhaust your power quickly. Focusing on multiple habits makes it impossible to maintain this strength over a long period of time and what usually happens is that you will give up once it becomes too difficult to change this routine.

During my weight loss journey, God helped me change one habit at a time. I knew I didn't have the power to change myself and I am being incredibly honest here. I didn't realise that losing weight is linked to change and changing daily habits and then doing this consistently for a long time. God in His mercy enabled me and began to do most of the habit changes from the inside out. The book of **Proverbs 22:6, NKJV** says,

> *"Train up a child in the way he should go, and when he is old, he will not depart from it."*

Often when we have made up our mind to lose weight, we are a like children who don't really know their left from right, and we need to be trained either through the help of a weight loss coach, nutritionist, dietician, or whichever path you choose to follow. You need to be trained to know what type of food to eat, what your portions should be like, why you need to start reading your food labels, why exercise is important, what you need to eat more of e.g. good fat instead of bad fat. You need to learn all of the things mentioned above and even more. Furthermore, you will need to start applying your new found knowledge consistently to see the desired result on your journey. This is why it is ideal to replace bad habits with good habits on your weight loss journey, then you will see permanent change.

Why Focus on One Habit at a Time?

A change of a single habit can help you develop a daily routine on your weight loss journey. For instance, once you have decided to lose weight a good daily habit would be to start eating a healthy breakfast two to three times a week. You can then proceed to four to five times a week, then finally making it seven days and that eventually becomes a habit. The important thing is to start small. It's unrealistic to start off with a plan to eat a healthy breakfast every day for 30 days. You will feel overwhelmed and will probably stop following this routine after a few days.

By focusing on a single habit at a time, you're able to create a lasting change in your routine. It's easier to maintain this new routine instead of trying to juggle multiple actions at the same time.

How to Form One Habit at a Time

The best way to make a permanent change is to focus on a single habit at a time. Here is a six-step process for getting started:

1. Identify What You Want To Change

You don't know what to change unless you put your finger on it. For me I wanted to change from being an emotional eater into a stable eater – one whose eating habits are not ruled by their emotions. That was the end goal, but I started by learning how to eat a healthy breakfast first. The habit I ought to develop is eating a healthy breakfast seven days a week, but I started with eating a healthy breakfast 3 to 5 times a week, then moved it to 7 days gradually.

2. Know Why You Are Doing It

If you don't know why you're doing it, then it will be less likely that you will follow through with the habit at all. This will decrease motivation. You can write down the reasons why you'd like to start eating a healthy breakfast. Is it to have more energy in the morning? Is it because you want your moods and emotions to be stable? Is it because you want to lose weight and you know eating breakfast will aid your weight loss journey? Write it down, whatever that reason may be, if it is not written down and carefully mapped out, it is only a wish or desire rather than a plan.

Once it is written down, look over it each day to remind yourself repeatedly. You might even choose to write on post-it notes and stick them around your house, on your bathroom mirror, your fridge door, on your laptop, on your wardrobe door or on your car dashboard. These reminders serve as a mirror each day. Always remember you will become like what you surround yourself with daily.

3. Identify the Bad Habit and Make a Substitute for It

If you don't find a substitute for the bad habit, it's easy to go right back to it after you've started to change it for a short time.

Going back to the healthy breakfast example, the bad habit would be not eating breakfast at all or eating food high in fat, sugar, and salt for breakfast. So, in order to change them, you would have to find a substitute for whatever you eat for breakfast in the morning e.g. oats with chopped banana to sweeten it or omelette with some salad, homemade granola with some yoghurt, yoghurt with fruit or a homemade green smoothie.

4. Stack up Your Chances for the Small Wins

You must make it as difficult for yourself as possible to retreat and go back to your bad habits. Using the same *eating habits example, identify and clean out your kitchen of all the bad foods that are lingering around. Replace them with healthy food, fruits, and veggies, and choose a cleaner eating lifestyle. Do the same for your desk at work or anywhere you have control over the environment. By doing this, you are setting yourself up to win. This will set you up for the small wins on your way to losing weight which is your main goal.*

5. Start the Process of Changing the Habit

Now since you've started the steps to prepare for the change, now it's time to make the change. Create a daily metric for tracking this change and start the habit immediately. Get an accountability group, choose to log it into a fitness app, and get your family and friends to keep you accountable. You need a support system; they are often your biggest cheerleaders on this journey.

6. Motivate by Giving Yourself a Reward Afterwards

Reward Yourself

Do you know that rewarding yourself is an important part of forming a new habit? Rewarding your newly developed (good) habits with something positive will encourage you to repeat the habits. It can help keep you motivated and on track, but it is important to do it the right way. It is important to remember we are rewarding the behaviour rather than the outcome. In this case, weight loss is an outcome of changing your eating and activity behaviour. Therefore, it is this behaviour we need to reinforce changing, which will in turn result in the weight loss. For example, if you have made a positive change to your meal pattern by eating regular healthy meals or eating healthy breakfast etc, this is a great thing to reward, whether you lose weight or not. It is also important to come up with a reward that is meaningful and relevant to you. It could be something as simple as setting aside time at the end of the week for a long indulgent bubble bath or an hour to watch your favourite sport TV.

Avoiding Food Rewards is Essential

A common misconception is that you had a great week making healthy choices and achieving your exercise goal, so you can treat yourself to a favourite food or a few drinks. After all, you have been so diligent all week it won't hurt, will it? It will.

Why is this unhelpful? Why should we avoid food rewards?

This kind of thinking can set you up for comfort eating. Often a single incidence of overeating is closely followed by another. "Oh well, I overate last night, and I ate the whole block of chocolate this morning, so I may as well continue." Remember, it is important to keep planning non-food rewards for non-achievements and achievements on your journey and after.

Example of Rewards

- Buying yourself a magazine/a bunch of flowers/some music/new trainers or workout gear.
- Getting a massage or a pedicure and manicure.
- Learn a new skill – Try playing the piano, singing, acting, or painting.
- Going on a skiing, snowboarding or beach vacation.
- Allocating time to do an activity you enjoy, a 'me-time' activity e.g. read a book or relax in a way you enjoy.
- Going out with a friend or treating yourself with a trip to the cinema/art gallery/ sports match, somewhere you will enjoy visiting.
- If you successfully include breakfast every day, you could reward yourself by putting aside a small amount of money on a weekly basis to buy yourself a nice new breakfast set – something nice to remind you of the benefits of consuming a healthy breakfast regularly.
- Asking your partner to take the kids out for the afternoon so you can enjoy a

empty house without interruptions.

Declutter your Life: "Seun, I am reading your book so that I can lose weight, why re you talking about decluttering?" Unfortunately, a cluttered house and mind is inked to weight gain. Let us define clutter first so that you begin to assess your ituation and see if this is one place that you need to start working on first before ny others.

The **Merriam Webster** Dictionary defines **'clutter'** as

To run in disorder.

To fill or cover with scattered or disordered things that impede movement or reduce effectiveness.

A collection of things lying about in an untidy state.

A crowded or confused mass or collection.

We can see from the descriptions above that clutter is when we have disorder in n area or all areas of our life. During my weight loss journey, this was one place n my life the Holy Spirit highlighted for me to work on, and as I began to work on t, it was as if dead weights were lifted from my life. I was very, very lazy, and I vould give excuses for not doing so many things, my mind was filled with junk, ny thought life was nothing to write home about. I believed whatever anyone old me about myself.

was a shopaholic who would buy on impulse and buy things I didn't need. I had every colour of shoes and bags, from green to red to yellow (there's absolutely 1othing in purchasing different shoes of different colours if your life is in order). When it came to make up, I was always buying the latest make up palette in town, always on to the next new lipstick that was reigning; meanwhile I was going into really bad debt. My wardrobe was full of an array of clothes I needed, and I didn't 1eed. Even where I was living, my room was untidy. I would wash clothes and leave them in the washing machine, to take them out and spread them on a drye was a problem. My flatmate at the time was always reprimanding me about i Once the clothes were dry, instead of folding them and putting them away, would just leave them on the bed where I would sleep with them until furthe notice.

The truth was that my mind and my environment were always in a mess. It i impossible to achieve anything with that type of mind-set, environment, an lifestyle. This was the main reason I often felt stressed, overwhelmed, an procrastinated a lot. I basically gave up on myself and life. The word of God say in the book of **1 Corinthians 14: 33, NIV**

"For God is not a God of disorder but of peace."

This scripture shows us the nature of God. God is not a God of clutter but c peace! Peace meaning calmness, order, stillness, and tranquillity. God loves yo right now whether you live in a clutter or not. His love for you will never chang and it is not based on your works, so be rest assured in that truth.

What clutter can do to you, however, is prevent you from experiencing the typ of life that Jesus died for you to enjoy because of your disorderly state of bein and environment. Have you noticed that we often hear God more when ou minds are not cluttered? Our minds are more alert and sharper when w exercise, because it helps to reduce stress and releases the 'feel good' hormone dopamine, which calms and makes us feel good. When you reduce your adde sugar intake and increase your vegetable intake, you tend to feel a lot bette lighter and at peace with yourself. Why? These things help you to declutter you mind and life, and in return help you to feel better.

Study after study has shown that clutter contributes to stress, anxiety, an depression. What you might not know, is that clutter contributes to weight gair

Here's how that happens.

In the book **_The Stress Solution_** by Arthur P. Ciaramicoli, an American psychologist, he explains how this works from a scientific perspective. The main issue is stress, which has myriad negative effects.

A recent study from the University of Zurich discovered that even moderate stress changes the brain chemistry that influences self-control. For the study, they had participants take an ice bath, which produced a moderate amount of stress. Those participants chose to eat unhealthy foods, demonstrating that when we are stressed, we seek comfort from foods that are sweet or high in fat. Cortisol (the "stress" hormone) causes our bodies to hold onto fat. This initiates a vicious cycle where our feelings of satiety (being full) are altered, our metabolism is slowed, and we crave more sugary and fatty foods.

Stress hormones have also been linked to inflammation. A study in the UK in 2008 showed a linear correlation with inflammation and weight gain. As inflammation increased, so did weight.

A cluttered kitchen environment has been shown to contribute to higher calorie consumption and unhealthy food choices.

The more I learn about decluttering and organising, the more I am astounded at how many areas of our lives are affected by clutter. If you've been trying to lose weight and have had no luck, your environment may be sabotaging your efforts. That means if you want to lose weight, you MUST change your environment, and that starts with decluttering your home.

During my journey, one of the many excuses I gave God was that where I was living was small and I remember the Lord correcting me while I was studying my Bible. I came across these words in the book of **Luke 16: 10, NLT**

"If you are faithful in little things, you will be faithful in large ones. But if you are dishonest in little things, you won't be honest with greater

responsibilities."

God corrected me that in order for Him to move me to a bigger place, I needed t
be faithful in tidying up the one I was presently living in and my perceptio
changed immediately, and I obeyed.

Until you declutter, all that clutter is going to keep causing stress (whether yo
realise it or not). Your self-control will be inhibited. Your desire to eat unhealth
foods will increase. Your metabolism will slow down. Decluttering and losin
weight have one huge thing in common – creating awareness. Once you are full
aware of what you're consuming and the impact of food on your body, it become
important to you to feed your body with the right food. When you consistentl
stay aware of the benefits of eating healthy, several things happen: you los
weight naturally and permanently, your energy levels rise and breed yet mor
motivation to continue, and niggling health problems often disappear
essentially decluttering further negativity from your life. Not only that, weigh
loss and decluttering tend to work in perfect harmony together, eac
encouraging the other.

The good news is that when your home starts to look more pleasing and whe
your routines and systems start to run smoothly, it's only natural that your min
will turn its attention to other areas which you might want to change. Likewis
when you're losing weight by intentionally making healthy choices, you see tha
you can make intentional choices within your home too. You start realisin
you're in the driving seat of your life and all you need to do is decide where yo
want it to go. Essentially, when you're making the decision that the only thing
entering both your home and body are going to nourish and add value, you'r
respecting yourself.

You can start by decluttering your kitchen one item at a time, one cupboard at
time; then move to your bedroom repeating the same process, and slowl

moving from each area of your house until you are done. By just dedicating five minutes a day, a whole lot of decluttering can be achieved in a week or a month. You never can tell; this could be the golden key to your weight loss journey. Start decluttering and don't over think it.

The Power of No: Nobody likes the idea of disappointing others but knowing when and how to say no is one of the most important skills you can cultivate. It is a learned act with the help of the Holy Spirit. Done right, "no" can help you build better relationships and free you up to do the things that are important to you.

Saying no was also one of my many weak points because I wanted to please people all the time, I found it hard to say no. The Holy Spirit highlighted this to me one day during my prayer time. I had another light bulb moment. I noticed that each time I said no to people, I was indirectly saying yes to myself. Each time I said no to more sleep in the morning, I was saying yes to spending more time with God. Each time I said no to unhealthy food, I was saying yes to healthy food. Each time I said no to buying what I didn't need, I was saying yes to my savings account and self-control. Each time I said no to procrastination, I was saying yes to discovering my ability. Each time I said no to a bad thought, I was saying yes to a good thought. Each time I said no to fear, I was saying yes to faith. Each time I said no to my comfort zone, I was learning to walk by faith and not sight. Each time I said no to a bottle of coke, I was saying yes to drinking water. I discovered that the power of 'No' was within me. The more I said no, the more my life was in order because of one little word – NO! I began to experience peace of mind, good health, and joy like never before.

During this time of learning, I found out that I was no longer feeling overwhelmed all the time and I wasn't feeling anxious either. Most people didn't like it because I was becoming a new person. A friend during that time asked me if I could help her list some things on eBay because I had already started selling my old clothes and shoes. I told her no, but I also told her I was willing to teach her by helping her set up her account. She wasn't happy about it, but I was able to help her set up her own account which paid off as she has had many sales through her own platform. If I hadn't said 'no' and taught her instead, she would have been dependent on me to help her list her products, sell them, and post them; and with my present situation I would not be able to fulfil that obligation.

Here are some ways to start building your ability to say that difficult word 'No'.

Acknowledge That You Can't Do Everything

Trying to say yes to everything is likely to leave you trapped with no time or energy for yourself or for the thing God has for you to do (and that was my life), and unable to give your best to any of your commitments.

I was guilty of this; I wasn't a committed person to anything, and the reason was that I was overcommitted to too much. I would often wake up and choose not to go for anything I was committed to. I gained a bad reputation with people. It was only during my weight loss journey that I realised this, and I started making wise decisions carefully and allowing the Holy Spirit to help me with this weakness. I discovered that I couldn't do everything for everyone and knowing that was a freedom in itself. I started by selecting the things I genuinely wanted to say yes to—taking my health seriously, choosing to save more money, the things that would build relationships with important people in my life, that aligned with Godly values, things that bring me joy and I stopped accepting responsibilities that didn't meet those criteria. Acknowledging I couldn't do everything, and I couldn't be everything to everybody really helped me, I am still on this journey because our lives are in season, so I often ask God what He wants me to say yes or no to.

Define Your Personal Boundaries

Defining your personal boundaries can be a very difficult thing to do initially if you are a people pleaser, with the help of God however, it becomes easier. Boundaries define the emotional and mental space between yourself and another person. I think of boundaries as the gatekeepers of my personal space and make sure that I'm clear about how much I can take on.

While I was writing this book, I was given just a few days' notice to attend an impromptu birthday celebration and a conference. Now the old me would have automatically said yes but I had to think it through because I currently have a lot on my plate. I had already planned that I would be using the weekend to write my book then I was invited to this celebration and conference at the last minute. I had to decide with the help of the Holy Spirit because I know the current season, I am in. I had to refuse because I knew the birthday celebrant was going to have another celebration in the summer. I also declined the invitation to the conference because I know there will be many more conferences that I can attend in the future. With that being said, setting boundaries, especially with people you care about, can be difficult and may make you feel guilty at first. Remember that caring for yourself helps assure that you have the energy to be there for others and with the help of the Holy Spirit setting boundaries becomes easier and easier each day.

Identify Your Priorities

The **Macmillan** Dictionary defines the word *'priority'* as something <u>important</u> that must be done first or <u>needs</u> more <u>attention</u> than anything else.

To make good decisions about what to say no to, you need a clear idea of your own priorities. The Holy Spirit helped me to begin to walk this path. I knew that spending time with God, exercising and meal prepping, was important to me and I began to prioritise them. Once I began to name and identify what was important to me each day by writing them down the night before, it made my decision-making process easier. My advice is to sit down and spend some time thinking about what's most important to you in this current season of your life and write them out. Learning to prioritise effectively can help you become more efficient, save time, and decrease stress. Once you know what's most important, it's easier to decide where to focus your energy.

Practice Saying the Words

Whether you're declining an invitation to a party, conference or turning down a new project at work, you can say no while still being friendly and respectful. Saying the word 'No' can feel rude at times especially if you are on the receiving end and you expect someone to turn up for you and support you. Over the years I have learnt to say, "Let me get back to you." By saying that it gives me enough time to check my calendar and see if I don't have anything planned on the day or to see how I can move things around to accommodate the request. Give yourself some ground rules and practice what you could say. You can give replies like "Can I get back to you", "Let me check my calendar" and after you have given these responses, you can then say 'No' in regard to the request. The truth is that some requests will warrant a 'No' on the spot because you already know that the day or time is not going to work out because of other commitments you may have. Always remember to give a brief reason if you wish to, but don't falter or back down. Be direct – "I'm sorry, but that's not something I can take on now."

Know That You Can't Please Everyone

Trying to make everyone happy is a recipe for stress and frustration, and it's literally impossible to do. You are not designed to make everybody happy, even Jesus Christ didn't make everyone happy. I lived with this mind-set (thinking that I could please everyone) for a very long time. I truly wanted to be everything to everybody, but I soon found out, that only God can fill that position. This desire drove me to a lot of stress at work and at home; the result was frustration which meant I resorted to food for comfort. I had to learn through the help of the Holy Spirit, that it was not my job to make everyone happy. I do care about people, but I will not allow anyone to put me on a guilt trip to make them happy.

You may fear that people will disrespect you or be disappointed if you say no but most people won't think any less of you. Remember too that in saying no you're modelling good self-care to those around you.

Here's the bottom line, knowing when to say no takes learning. Hone your skills so that you're able to more easily recognise and deal with the situations where it's your best response.

Nuggets For A Healthy Lifestyle

Eat Breakfast: There is so much news and controversy these days about eating breakfast or not. One school of thought says, breakfast is the most important meal of the day, another school of thought says it's not. Who are we to believe? What I do know from my personal journey and as a coach who helps people to embrace a healthy lifestyle, is that breakfast is important just like other meals are too. Breakfast is considered an important meal because it breaks the overnight fasting period, replenishes your supply of glucose, and provides other essential nutrients to keep your energy levels up throughout the day. Lots of people talk about the benefits of breakfast and the science that backs it up too. Research shows that people who eat breakfast are:

- Less likely to be overweight than those who skip breakfast.
- Able to concentrate for longer and have better memory and problem-solving skills.
- More likely to get the right amount of vital nutrients (such as calcium and B vitamins) than people who skip breakfast.
- Likely to consume less saturated fat and have lower levels of unhealthy cholesterol.
- Eating healthy and nutritious breakfast reduces risk of starving as well as craving or overeating throughout the day.

- A morning meal helps keep your blood sugar stable.
- Eating a healthy breakfast helps you feel fuller for longer and eat fewer calories throughout the day thus helping to control your weight.

Breakfast is as important as all the other meals you have during the day, when you eat a healthy breakfast, it sets you up for success on your weight loss journey.

I had to learn to start eating a healthy breakfast and it was a journey. I soon noticed that once I had a healthy breakfast, my mood was very stable, and I was able to concentrate for a longer period of time; and I didn't feel tired like I use to. If you do not have a breakfast routine, it is likely that you don't roll out of the bed and fancy food. The thought of food at that time might even make you feel a bit nauseated. However, scientists know that an erratic eating pattern can make our hunger and fullness sensations unreliable signals of when to eat. The good news is that you can get those signals working again (to feel hungry in the morning) by adjusting your body clock. To do this, start with simple breakfast options like a piece of fruit or a pot of yoghurt. Then build from this to form new habits.

On my journey, I had to research on healthy breakfast ideas to help me embrace this new lifestyle. Below are some examples of breakfast food items you can start incorporating into your meals.
- High fibre or wholegrain cereal – Oats, Weetabix, homemade granola with skimmed milk, greek or plant base yoghurt with any fruit of your choice.
- Mix fresh fruits (see what is in season) with greek, natural, plant base yogurt. You can add some protein like chia seeds, mixed seed, linseed, hemp seed to it.
- Smoothies – Blend water with 1.5 cup of spinach, 1 stick of celery stick, 1/2 medium size orange, 1 medium size kiwi, 1/3 cucumber,1/2 avocado, a little ginger and 1 teaspoon of chia seed.
- Boiled, poached, or scrambled egg with tomato, spinach and mushroom or

any vegetable of your choice.

Pancakes made with wholemeal flour topped with fruit compete.

Wholegrain or Wholemeal bread with egg or avocado and some vegetables like tomatoes, cucumber etc

Boiled semi ripe plantain with scrambled egg or with vegetable stew.

No one starts a new lifestyle that is automatic from the beginning, the best approach is to take it one day at a time and be open to trying something you have never tried before. Breakfast is just as important as any other meal.

Eat Whole Food or Real Food: The closer you eat food made from the earth, the easier your weight loss journey becomes. Eating healthy, non-processed, fresh, whole food – real food, was a total game change for me. Put simply, real food is food as it is found in nature (single-ingredient foods are best, as are unprocessed, unaltered foods made without any chemicals or additives). Real food is food that nourishes our bodies and minds with vitamins and minerals and makes us feel good after we eat it. Real food is food that improves our health, not destroys it. Real food is medicine to our bodies, making them better!

What we see in most supermarket aisles is not real food. Most of the food we see in glossy packaging have been refined and packed well to appeal to our human eyes. They are full of sugar, trans fats and refined carbohydrates, and one thing they have in common is that they will not keep you full for long. They are full of empty calories, you become addicted to them, they are quick and easy to get, and they often lead to chronic diseases and illnesses. I used to have painful menstrual cramps, rashes under my armpits, severe back pain, constant feelings of tiredness and bloating, severe mood swings, feelings of crankiness and my self-confidence was low. The month I started eating real food I began to see changes, and 95% of all the symptoms I complained of disappeared within six months.

I have also had numerous testimonies from residents of London Barking and

Dagenham whom I coach daily, that most ailments like migraines, high cholesterol, Type 2 diabetes, polycystic ovaries, asthma, hypertension, osteoarthritis, and rheumatoid arteritis, mostly disappear after a few months and they are feeling better than before. Reports like these help me know that when we feed our bodies with real food, we reap a reward of good health.

What does real food look like?

- Real foods are more a product of nature than a product of industry.
- Lots of fruits and vegetable (fresh or frozen or tinned)
- Dairy products like milk, unsweetened yoghurt, eggs, and cheese or plant base product.
- 100% whole-wheat and whole grains
- Lean meats such as pork, beef, chicken, turkey, and fish such as salmon, mackerel, tuna, sea bass, sardine, cod etc.
- Beverages limited to water, milk, all-natural juices, coffee & tea, and fruit teas.
- All-natural sweeteners including 100% organic honey and dates syrup are acceptable in moderation.

Eating Out and Partying: This was one area I found very challenging on my weight loss journey. At first, I turned down a lot of eating out and partying, because I just wanted to be focused and to get into the zone of losing weight. As I progressed on my journey, I found out I just couldn't avoid going out to eat and party because it was beyond my control. I realised that I just needed to be a lot wiser with my choices and decisions. Over the years, I have gotten smarter and smarter about eating out and partying. Always remember Rome was not built in a day, as you go along you will learn what not to eat, do and what you can do before you even step out.

Eating out can be a fun and enjoyable part of healthy living. If you know how to do it without upsetting your goal. It can be challenging but it is doable.

Below are some tips that will help you know what to do when you are eating out during and after your weight loss journey.

Things To Remember When Eating Out

. Before You Go

Go in with a game plan: Go on the restaurant's website to check the menu and nutritional information ahead of time, this will ensure you know what you are eating beforehand.

Have a healthy snack before you go: Never arrive at the restaurant hungry. If you do, you will eat anything that is offered. Try having a fruit, yoghurt with fruits, or dips and vegetable sticks.

Plan lighter meals: This balances out the fact that you are likely to eat more when you are out. If going for a dinner, you can decide to have a green smoothie for breakfast and have chicken and avocado salad for lunch. It all depends on how you wish to do the ratio.

Be more active: Do more physical activity on the days around eating out to help balance the extra energy you might consume.

. When You Arrive

Have a glass of water: This helps to fill you up before having any meal and it can also help you to avoid unnecessary liquid calories from other drinks just because you are thirsty. Choose sparkling water or still water as you prefer.

Choose free food wisely: Free foods are olives, nuts, breads, prawn crackers from the table and often they are free. You can ask the waiter to remove them or have one slice only and limit the oil or butter.

Placing Your Order

Have one or two out of the three: Instead of a starter, main meal, and desserts, choose a combination of one or two e.g. go for the starter and skip starter and desserts, or starter and main, or main and desert.

- Fill up on vegetables and salad: Most restaurants now serve vegetables and salad as extra side. You can choose to order and remember you can still follow the balanced meal plate too for portion control.

- Menu words to avoid: Avoid dishes that are fried, deep-fried, pan fried, breaded, battered, creamy, crispy, cheesy, au gratin, buttered, tempura etc.

- Spot the healthy choices: Choose lean meats and dishes that are grilled, steamed, baked, or stir fried (rather than fried). Don't be afraid to ask how the food is cooked, the waiters will gladly tell you.

- Never be afraid to ask: Whether it is less cheese on your pizza or the dressing you put on the side, ask the waiter. They are used to people making requests and speaking up could help you make the best choice for your weight loss goal.

- Sauces on the side: Ask for dressing, sauces, and gravies on the side, then you are in better control of how much fat you add to your meal.

- Dessert dos and don'ts: Choose fruit-based options if possible, for dessert and avoid adding extra fats such as cream or ice cream. If not just go for your main meals.

3. When You Are Eating

- Don't feel you have to finish your meal: Remember restaurants portions are big and there will be many other times you can eat those foods again. If others push you, have the confidence to say no.

- Prevent picking: Offer your leftovers to others, cover your plate or call the waiter to clear your plate.

Party Survival Guide

Parties are all about celebration and celebration often centre on food and drinks. They can seem challenging, especially as party foods and canapé trays are generally very high in fat and sugar.

However, being aware of your portion sizes and how to make healthier choices means you can stick to your goals while still having fun. Here are some ideas to help.

Avoid the buffet table: Fill your plate just once and don't go back for more. Always remember the balance meal plate ½ vegetables and the other ½ protein and carbs. Ask the Holy Spirit to help you exercise self-control.

Don't deny yourself: Eating healthy doesn't mean you have to avoid foods, just watch your portion sizes. Choose one or two favourites options form the buffet table rather than sampling them all.

Dance and Distract: Parties are about a lot more than food and drink. Learn new steps of dances, it is a fantastic way of burning more calories, make new friends also and before you know it, it is time to go home.

Always remember you can still eat out, party, and still lose weight; all you just need to do is be wise. The tips above can also be applied or used for unplanned meals and impromptu takeaways as well as pre planned events.

Treat Every Day Like A New Beginning: Start each day by affirming to yourself that you will do the best you can—no matter what happened yesterday. We often spend our time focusing on our past and we forget that our best days are still ahead. When we put our focus on our past, the devil loves it but when we keep pressing into our future, God will do exceedingly, abundantly and above all we could ever ask for. Psalm 118: 24, CEV says

"This day belongs to the LORD! Let's celebrate and be glad today."

The Lord has blessed us, with a brand-new day and we ought to be celebrating – being glad in it. Start seeing each day as an opportunity, a gift from God and a fresh start.

Love Yourself: Loving yourself can be hard even before starting or during your weight loss journey. It can be hard if you have had lots of negative words sown into your life which often lead you to not believing much in yourself or can lead to you comparing yourself to others. In the past, loving myself was hard, but it was during my weight loss journey, that the Lord began to teach me how I needed to accept who He had created me to be whether I got to my desired goal or not. The truth is that I never really loved myself, I grew up not believing much in myself. I was often compared to others and as a result I never felt I was worthy of anything since I believed other people were better than me. These negative beliefs impacted my life so much and my life revolved around them. The world we live in doesn't help either because if you don't know who you are, the world will tell you what you are not, based on its value system and belief system.

One day while I was studying the book of **Genesis 1:31,** NLT

"Then God looked over all he had made, and he saw that it was very good! And evening passed and morning came, marking the sixth day."

The Bible says, *'very good',* another translation says it was excellent. Good means excellent, of high quality, satisfactory in quality, pleasant to look at, giving lots of value, advantageous, best. This is what God says about you and me! Whether you are big, tall, fat, slim, healthy, or unhealthy right now God says you are good. God loves you whether you lose weight or not. Losing weight or changing your lifestyle to be healthier will enable you to have a body that is energised, and you will be able to carry out your purpose on earth effectively.

This truth began a healing process in my soul and the more I saw myself the way God saw me, the more I was ready to accept and value myself more by nourishing my body with the right food. Always remember you are a work in progress, Jesus died for you, He was crucified, buried, and raised to a new life because of you – you are worth dying for. When we take in the word of God and know that He loves us unconditionally, our weight loss journey and life after it becomes easier.

Love yourself, you will never get another you. It might not be the easiest thing in the world to do, but it's the most important.

Learn To Give Yourself Compliments: It may sound silly, but it can help encourage self-kindness to come naturally (and limit self-doubt, which can lead to self-loathing). Remembering what you love about yourself puts you in the right mind-set to want the best for your body. I had to learn this during my journey. After a good workout, I will give myself a verbal pat on the back by saying "Well done." When I put on an outfit, I will tell myself "Seun you look good." Once I clean my house and it looks good, I pat myself at the back.

I realised that the more I did this, the more I began to feel good about myself and all the words of negativity began to leave. Don't wait for others to compliment you on your weight loss journey or after, choose to compliment yourself each day and if others do it, it is a bonus.

Stop Comparing Yourself to Others: The Bible says in **2 Corinthians 10: 12, CEV:**

"We won't dare compare ourselves with those who think so much of themselves. But they are foolish to compare themselves with themselves."

The Bible says when we compare ourselves with others, we are foolish, meaning we are unwise and lacking good sense. I used to compare myself with other people so much that I didn't even know who I was and never had a relationship with myself. Can you imagine waking up and always thinking someone is better than you and wanting their life? Well guess what, thinking like that will lead you into hatred, jealousy, envy, and strife – all these things are the works of the flesh. **Galatians 5: 19-21, GW** says,

"Now, the effects of the corrupt nature are obvious: illicit sex, perversion, promiscuity, idolatry, drug use, hatred, rivalry, jealousy, angry outbursts,

selfish ambition, conflict, factions, envy, drunkenness, wild partying, and similar things. I've told you in the past and I'm telling you again that people who do these kinds of things will not inherit God's kingdom."

Once I knew that those were the works of the flesh and I no longer had that nature in me, I had to learn to work and live by the fruits of the spirit – it brought me life and peace. **Galatians 5: 22 – 23, NLT** says,

"But the Holy Spirit produces this kind of fruit in our lives: love, joy, peace, patience, kindness, goodness, faithfulness, gentleness, and self-control. There is no law against these things!"

Comparisons can make you feel bad about yourself. What is the point of that? You are unique, you are one of a kind, you are precious, you are God's workmanship, you are valued by God and you are the apple of God's eye. Start believing the best of yourself and comparison will be killed for life. Focus on your unique talents and being the best version of who God created you to be.

Set Attainable Goals: Aiming to drop a dress size in time for a friend's birthday party in six days, is an easy path to disappointment and self-blaming or aiming to lose over 20 kgs in two to three months will result in the same self-blame. Moreover, coming down on yourself in this way can contribute to increased levels of the stress hormone cortisol, which has been shown to increase the amount of belly fat stored by the body, particularly in women.

Setting a more attainable goal, such as trying a new exercise class once a week, eating breakfast five days a week or swapping one sweet treat for a healthier option, is a better way to protect your self-esteem and respect your body's limits. Why set attainable goals? It is all about motivation. Knowing you are taking steps towards achieving a goal is rewarding and gives you something to work towards. What's more, behaviour change experts recommend goal setting as one of the most effective ways to change your behaviour and develop new healthier habits. It is all about ensuring your goals are SMART (Specific, Measurable, Achievable, Relevant, Time specific).

- **Specific** – *I will eat a healthy lunch every day rather than I will eat healthy.*
- **Measurable** – *I will do 300 minutes of activity a week rather than I will do more exercise.*
- **Achievable** – *I will limit myself to two pieces of rich tea biscuits twice a week rather than I will cut out biscuits.*
- **Relevant** – *YOUR GOALS should be personal to you, there is no point cutting back on biscuits if you only eat them occasionally anyway.*
- **Time specific** – *Set realistic, short-term time frames e.g. I will exercise on three days next week, rather than I will exercise three days a week.*

Using the SMART approach on your weight loss journey, will keep you on track and make it much easier to form new habits that will help you lose weight and keep the weight off.

Believe What God Says About You: The more we see ourselves through the eyes of God, the more we love ourselves. Often the reason so many of us never love ourselves or believe the best of ourselves is because first of all, we don't even know what God says about us. Secondly, we never really had the right people to affirm to us or call out the best in us. Loving yourself is equal to believing the best of what God says you are. We must learn to separate our 'who' from our 'do' and many of us don't know what that is. Our 'who' is who God says we are and that can only be found through Christ Jesus (your identity) and it is permanent and unchangeable. Our 'do' is our behaviour, attitude, jobs, where we live etc. Who we are is fixed and never changing in Christ Jesus, but what we do will continually change from one level of glory to another as we renew our mind to the word of God? Learn to believe what God says about you and keep pressing on. The scriptures below emphasizes this.

2 Corinthians 5: 17, ESV

"Therefore, if anyone is in Christ, he is a new creation. The old has passed away; behold, the new has come."

1 Peter 2: 9, ESV

"But you are a chosen race, a royal priesthood, a holy nation, a people for his own possession, that you may proclaim the excellencies of him who called you out of darkness into his marvellous light."

Ephesians 2: 10, ESV

"For we are his workmanship, created in Christ Jesus for good works, which God prepared beforehand, that we should walk in them."

Reflect On The Gifts Your Body Has Given You: Your body has carried you through all the seasons of life and you should appreciate it. It could be that it propelled you through your half marathon, it gave you two beautiful children, maybe you had an accident, or you were sick, and your body healed perfectly; while you were underweight or overweight this body helped you to accomplish your day-to-day tasks. The body that you may be down on has undoubtedly brought you great opportunity and joy. *Revelling in those experiences* and all that are still in store for you is an important way to love yourself while you lose weight or build a much healthier lifestyle.

Work on Your Stress Levels: Feeling pressured and anxious are other factors we might not recognise that foil our efforts to lose and keep off weight. Stress increases comfort eating – our desire to consume foods that make us feel better emotionally. Unfortunately, most of us don't reach for a fresh salad and a nice piece of salmon or healthier snacks. Refined carbs, saturated fats, salty and sweet nacks are more a typical go-to for people under pressure. Stress also triggers the elease of <u>cortisol</u> in the body, which leads to higher insulin levels and, in turn, veight gain (especially dangerous <u>belly fat</u>). Worse still, the combination of ortisol and high-fat, high-sugar foods appear to interfere with leptin, one of the ormones that helps regulate your appetite. As you well know, anxiety and stress an keep you from getting the restorative sleep you need to maintain a healthy veight.

One way to manage stress at mealtimes is to be aware of your stress triggers. Over he years, I have learnt to be aware of situations that will normally put me in a tressful position and learnt how to overcome them through the help of the Holy pirit. A scripture that comes to mind is **Philippians 4: 6-7, NLT** which says,

"*Don't worry about anything; instead, pray about everything. Tell God what you need and thank him for all he has done. Then you will experience God's peace, which exceeds anything we can understand. His peace will guard your hearts and minds as you live in Christ Jesus.*"

remember I was shocked when I came across this scripture. I couldn't believe hat God was telling me not to worry about anything. I was a worrier by default, nd I would worry about so many things that would never happen. Over the ears, I have learnt to trust God with my life, and it still is an ongoing process. earning to trust God will take time, but the more you learn to do it by praying nd going to Him at all times and not only when circumstances that warrant vorry or stress come, it becomes easier and easier. The best antidote for worry or tress is prayer. Worry and stress will not just vanish, but the answer is to pray bout the situation, entrusting that God is working on it. Part of loving yourself is earning to cast your cares on God, we were never designed to be stress-filled all he time.

Measure yourself: Scales don't always give you the whole story about your body or your weight loss progress, I had to learn that during my weight loss journey and began to look at different ways I can measure myself. For that reason, scales (when used alone) aren't the best way to track what's really going on inside and outside your body.

Another reason to avoid using only scales is the emotional nature of weighing ourselves. Stepping on a scale doesn't just give us a number, it can determine how we feel about ourselves and this affects our body image, which in turn can make your weight loss journey miserable. The problem with bodyweight scales is that they measure everything — fat, muscle, bones, organs and even that sip of water or bite of food you've had. The scale can't tell you what you've lost or gained, which is important information if you're trying to lose weight—and by weight, what we really mean is fat.

How Can I Be Proactive About Measuring Myself?
1) Take Your Body Measurements
One of the different ways to measure yourself is by tracking progress because it doesn't require any fancy equipment, and anyone can do it. Taking your measurements at certain areas can give you an idea of where you are losing fat, which is important since we all lose fat in different areas and in a different order. Taking your measurements can help reassure you that things are happening—even if you're not losing fat exactly where you want just yet and it saves you from being frustrated all the time.

When measuring, start by wearing tight-fitting clothing (or no clothing) and make a note of what you're wearing so you know to wear the same clothes the next time you measure. Here's how to do it:

- **Bust:** Measure around the chest right at the nipple line, but don't pull the tape too tight.
- **Chest:** Measure just under your bust.
- **Waist:** Measure a half-inch above your belly button or at the smallest part of

your waist.

- **Hips:** Place the tape measure around the biggest part of your hips.
- **Thighs:** Measure around the biggest part of each thigh.
- **Calves:** Measure around the largest part of each calf.
- **Upper arm:** Measure around the largest part of each arm above the elbow.
- **Forearm:** Measure around the largest part of the arm below the elbow.

Take them again once a month to see if you're losing inches, which of course you will lose.

2) How Your Clothes Fit

Another simple way to track progress is how your clothes fit. You may want to take a picture of yourself wearing a bathing suit, keep it in your weight loss journal. Each month take a new picture and you'll be surprised at how many changes you notice in a picture as opposed to just seeing yourself in the mirror. You can also use your clothes to keep track of your progress. Choose one pair of trousers, top or dress that are a little tight and try them on every four weeks to see how they fit. Make a note of where they feel loose, where they feel tight, and how you feel wearing them. Focusing on how your clothes fit may help boost self-esteem and inspire you to stick with your plan as opposed to being frustrated by a specific number on the scale.

3) Your Mood

When you fuel yourself with healthy foods and get enough physical activity, not only will you lose weight, but you will also start to feel better mentally. This is my story, the moment I started eating healthy and getting physically active, my moods changed drastically. You might have to learn how to look away from the scale for a while and just focus on how you feel. Do you have more energy? Do you look forward to the day? Are you learning to love and respect your body? In my Lean Living sessions, I have discovered that most people will not really see drastic change in weight loss at the beginning and that is why I always ask them how they feel. Most times I hear 'I am sleeping better', 'I feel lighter', 'My moods are more stable, and my cholesterol is going down'.

The better your moods, the easier it is to stick with the healthy eating habit, even if you have not noticed lots of changes, and that will also build your self-confidence to keep going.

4) Your Strength

If you didn't get much physical activity before you embarked on your weight-loss journey but you're maintaining a regular exercise regimen today, you're probably able to push yourself further than before. An increase in strength is an indirect measure of weight loss and it's also an empowering reminder that you're getting into shape through your own hard work. Track how much further you can walk, run, cycle or swim, or how much longer you're active for compared to the previous day, previous week or previous month. As your health and fitness improves, you should be able to speak and breathe easier at the given activity level.

5) Your Sleep

You may notice you've been getting better quality sleep lately because of your positive lifestyle changes. Not only is sleep tied to weight loss, it also helps you stay healthy overall by reducing inflammation, helping repair muscles, reducing stress levels and allowing you to perform your best when exercising.

Enjoy the journey: With all the above being said and done. You will have to learn to enjoy every single day of losing weight, living a healthy lifestyle, clearing your debt, and discovering yourself. Always remember Rome was not built in a day. Learning to enjoy each day will set you up for success, it is a thing of the mind. Life is full of so many surprises and challenges, only those who have predetermined to keep going whether the going gets tough or not are able to stay on top of their goals. Things will get tough but with the help of the Holy Spirit and eeing your circumstances through the eyes of faith, you will be victorious. Make up your mind today and choose to enjoy the journey.

) Start each day with God

Ensure you start each day with God in prayer and studying the word. Having quiet time with God is a vital, it is a need and not a want. Spending time with God will help you to be more discerning on your journey and help you overcome so many challenges you will encounter on the way. Always remember you will become like the person you move with regularly. If you want to become more loving, self-controlled, full of hope and faith, stable and relentless; then take time out each day and spend it with your maker, the journey will be much easier. God will empower you to overcome whatever challenges you may face on your journey.

) Celebrate Every Small Win

It is so easy to be obsessed about the destination that we miss out on the journey. Make time to — celebrate your winsno matter how small. If you lose a few pounds or kilo, your clothes feel better, you sleep well or you are drinking more water, eating more vegetables or fruits, celebrate it (not with food). If you pay off some of your debts, celebrate it. What you celebrate will become bigger and bigger.

) Trust The Process

Life is not a 100-metre dash, it is a marathon. You have a long way to go on your weight lose journey so trust the process, it is leading you somewhere and the process is making you stronger; it is building you form the inside out, it is turning you into an overcomer.

) Make Time for Gratitude and Appreciation

Take time out and practice gratitude and appreciation. What you focus on will become your reality. The mere fact that you are alive is something to be grateful for. Start a gratitude journal and see after 30 days what you have written down, you will be grateful. Show me a person that is full of gratitude and I will show you a person who has chosen to enjoy life no matter what comes against them.

5) Spend Money on Experiences, Not Possessions

Experiences, not possessions create memories and meaning. Instead of having your wardrobe full of clothes, save that money and go on a trip with your friends or family. Take yourself on a solo holiday and experience what it feels like being you. Learn to create memories and not to acquire possessions.

6) Try New Things

Try something new that will challenge you, take up a new hobby. Try going to a sewing, soap making or cooking class. Start blogging or write your first book (like I am doing now) or start a business, whatever it is just try! You don't know where it will lead you and if you fail, pick up yourself and start again. You never know until you try, so make the effort and do something new.

7) Nurture Your Positive Relationships

Identify the people who lift you up and focus your energy on them. You will become like your circle. Look for people who will always see the best in you and see your potential. Ask God for help and He will grant you a spirit of discernment to choose your circle of friends, nurture such relationships.

8) Stay Positive

There is rarely any good news these days. When you turn on the TV or go to social media platforms, the vibe is often negative. Are these platforms bad? No, but you need to choose what enters your heart and mind daily, because as you think, so you become. Stay positive by meditating on the word of God and things that bring out the best in you. Save yourself energy and spend your time on things that are worthwhile.

9) Make Time to Relax or Rest

Making time to relax and reconnect with ourselves doesn't come naturally to us, but it is essential for the race of life. When you relax or rest, you are better equipped to deal with more challenging periods. Light a candle to relax, spend time with God, have a bubble bath, read a book, or bake your favourite treat. Resting is essential for your well-being.

10) Make Yourself a Priority

Putting yourself first by getting yourself healthy doesn't mean you don't care for others. Always remember a healthy you is a gift to your family and the world around you. Take time out to eat healthy and exercise regularly. The healthier you are, the better for yourself and more people will enjoy you.

11) Give Back to the Society

There is something about us that when we give to those who can't repay us, we get some form of fulfilment and joy back from it. We have been designed to look out for other people and to see how we can meet needs within our capacity. Give back by mentoring or coaching a teenager, choose to volunteer in your borough for a cause or support a charity by fund raising for them. Start small and see where it will lead you.

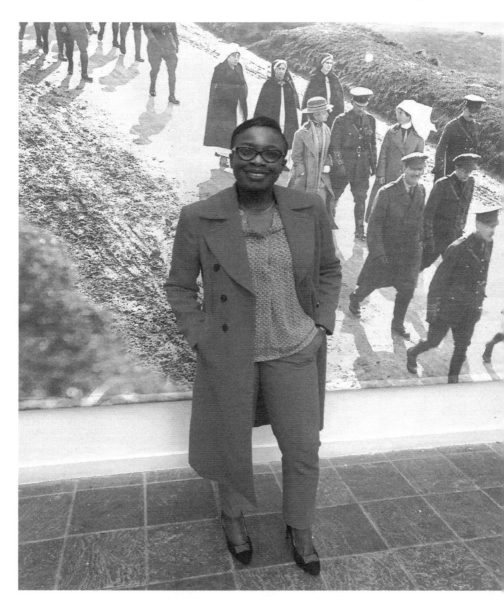

2019

You Can, You Will Because God Says So

Let me leave you with this note – You can, and you will lose weight, come out of debt, discover your passion/purpose, and you can overcome whatever challenge you are facing now because God says so. Isn't that reassuring knowing that you are not alone on this journey – knowing that your Heavenly Father will teach you, lead you, guide you, strengthen you, comfort you, reassure you, encourage you day in day out on this journey you are either in or about to embark on. This is why you need to get God involved so that you can come out victorious.

The book of **Philippians 1:6,** AMP says,

"I am convinced and confident of this very thing, that He who has begun a good work in you will [continue to] perfect and complete it until the day of Christ Jesus [the time of His return]."

Paul was the author of the book of Philippians and he wrote this letter to thank them for the work of financial partnership in advancing the good news (The gospel). He knew deep down in his heart that only God could have started that good work in them and only God could complete it and not man. Paul said, 'I am convinced and confident', what a bold statement to make. He knew based on his experiences with God, it was impossible for God to start something in one's life and not complete it.

The book of **Revelation 1:8, AMP** says,

"I am the Alpha and the Omega [the Beginning and the End]," says the Lord God Who is [existing forever] and Who was [continually existing in the past] and Who is to come, the Almighty [the Omnipotent, the Ruler of all]."

Whenever I read this passage I am encouraged, and my faith is stirred up. God is the Alpha and Omega of all things; He is the Beginning and End of all things

What a wonderful God we serve.

Remember that this journey is a good work He alone started in you. By reading this book, God has started a good work in you – the journey of living a healthy or balanced life, losing weight or overall well-being and He has reassured us that He alone will complete it as your partner with Him.

Be rest assured that I am rooting and clapping for you daily; and I am also praying for you because I know you will make it if you don't give up. If I can lose weight, get over depression, come out of huge debt, have a sound and disciplined mind, and be blessed in many other ways, you can too. You can because with God nothing is impossible.

Moving Forward

I am sure by now you have started working on the behaviours or habits you have listed in Books One and Two, which will aid and equip you to lose weight, or choose to start living a healthy/balanced lifestyle. I think it's necessary to remind you again at this stage that nothing happens until you make that decision or make up your mind, the truth is that no one can decide for you except you.

Now that you have decided to change your lifestyle, let us invite God in to lead and guide you on this journey.

Pray the prayer below:

Heavenly Father, I come to you today asking for your grace to commit to this new lifestyle change I am about to embark on/have started working on. I ask that you help me, lead me, guide me on this weight loss journey, coming out of debts, overcoming emotional issue, etc.. (Kindly list other things you want the Lord to help you overcome).

Heavenly Father, your word says, 'I can do all things through Christ who strengthens me' and I believe it with all my heart. Through your word Lord, I know I am not on this journey alone, because you are with me always to guide and encourage me when I feel like giving up. Thank you because you are the one that has begun this good work in me, and you will complete it. I know the journey will not be easy, but with you all things are possible. Thank you in advance for the victory I have over every single one of the issues I have brought before you. In Jesus name I pray. Amen

Now that we have invited God into this journey. The plan for action below has been designed to get you thinking on what areas in your weight loss journey or life changes need to happen, then begin to make those changes or reinforce the changes you have already started making from Books Two and Three. Take some time out and work through each one of them. Be very honest with the answers you give, remember once you identify the problem, you have already solved half of it.

1. Why do I want to change my eating habit, lose weight, or live a healthier/balanced lifestyle, or get of debt or...?

2. What made you make up your mind?

3. What are the top three areas you would like to start working on? E.g. Relationship with God, portion control, cut of sugar, start exercising, declutter my house etc.

1)

2)

3)

4. Which one of them is my top priority and why?

5. Have you prayerfully asked God for help or to show you the way to make this change?

6. When do you intend to start making the change or form new habits?

7. What plan for action have you put in place? E.g. Start exercising, start budgeting, wake up early in the morning to spend time with God, join a financial freedom class etc.

8. Working towards this goal is important to me because
....
....………….. E.g. it will help me to eat less sugar or exercise etc., which is good for my lifestyle change.

9. The plans I need to put in place to help me achieve my goals are:

10. Things that will stand in my way of achieving my goal are:

11. Solutions I could use to overcome these barriers are:

*This is just a reminder that you will face barriers and obstacles on your way to a better you, but there is always a way out with God.

12. I could get further support from.. E.g. Friends or Family or work colleagues etc.

13. Have you set a SMART goal? Choose one thing on the top three priority list mentioned above and start working on it. Focus on one thing and work through it repeatedly before you focus on the next one.

14. When are you going to review your goals?

1. Fortnightly

2. Monthly

3. Quarterly

"Everyone thinks of changing the world, but no one thinks of changing himself." - *Leo Tolstoy*. Remember you can do all things through Christ who strengthens you.

References

- www.matalan.co.uk (accessed December 2019)

- www.medicinenet.com (accessed May 2019)

- https://discovermomenta.com/ (accessed November 2019)

- https://jamesclear.com/new-habit (accessed May 2019)

- www.beateatingdisorders.org.uk (accessed May 2019)

- https://www.nhs.uk/live-well/ (accessed April 2019)

- https://blog.iqmatrix.com/a-life-of-excuses (accessed February 2020)

- https://blog.anytimefitness.com/395419-41-awesome-non-food-rewards-for-weight-loss (accessed June 2020)

- https://blog.myfitnesspal.com/5-motivating-ways-to-measure-loss-success/ (accessed November 2019)

- https://en.wikipedia.org/wiki/John_Stephen_Akhwari (accessed December 2020)

- https://icecreaminspiration.com/how-decluttering-helps-you-lose-weight/ (accessed October 2019)

- https://medicalxpress.com/news/2018-12-junk-food-diet-depression.html (accessed September 2019)

- https://thatsugarmovement.com/sugar-swaps/ (accessed September 2019)

- https://tlexinstitute.com/how-to-effortlessly-have-More-positive-thoughts (accessed December 2020)

- https://www.atidymind.co.uk/slim-your-life-slim-your-body/ (accessed June 2019)

- https://www.bbcgoodfood.com/howto/guide/how-much-water-should-i-drink-day (accessed October 2019)

References

- https://www.betterhealth.vic.gov.au/health/healthyliving/fruit-and-vegetables (accessed September 2019)

- https://www.bhf.org.uk/informationsupport/support/healthy-living/healthy-eating/salt (accessed February 2020)

- https://www.bulbanksmedicalcentre.co.uk/syndication/live-well/exercise/exercise-health-benefits (accessed December 2019)

- https://www.choosemyplate.gov/eathealthy/vegetables/vegetables-nutrients-health (accessed December 2019)

- https://www.crosswalk.com/faith/spiritual-life/7-Bible-figures-who-struggled-with-depression.html (accessed September 2019)

- Momenta – Your momenta handbook Page 71 – 73, 117 – 122, 202 – 204 (accessed February 2020)

- https://www.developgoodhabits.com/one-habit-at-a-time/ (accessed December 2019)

- https://www.diabete.qc.ca/en/living-with-diabetes/diet/tips-and-tricks/the-balanced-plate (accessed October 2019)

- https://www.gov.uk/government/publications/physical-activity-guidelines-uk-chief-medical-officers-report (accessed November 2019)

- https://www.health.harvard.edu/heart-health/the-sweet-danger-of-sugar (accessed November 2019)

- https://www.healthline.com/nutrition/10-benefits-of-exercise (accessed December 2019)

- https://www.healthline.com/nutrition/drinking-water-helps-with-weight-loss (accessed December 2019)

- https://www.heart.org/en/healthy-living/healthy-eating/eat-

References

smart/sugar/tips-for-cutting-down-on-sugar (accessed March 2020)

- https://www.heartfoundation.org.au/healthy-eating/food-and-nutrition/fats-and-cholesterol/monounsaturated-and-polyunsaturated-omega-3-and-omega-6-fats#balanceoffats (accessed January 2020)

- https://www.inc.com/lolly-daskal/stop-saying-yes-when-you-want-to-say-no.html (accessed October 2019)

- https://www.joe.co.uk/fitness-health/junk-food-depression-risk-212920 (accessed December 2020)

- https://www.mayoclinic.org/healthy-lifestyle/fitness/in-depth/exercise/art-20048389 (accessed February 2019)

- https://www.mayoclinic.org/healthy-lifestyle/nutrition-and-healthy-eating/in-depth/water/art-20044256 (accessed February 2019)

- https://www.medicalnewstoday.com/articles/319991.php#why-cut-out-sugar (accessed January 2020)

- https://www.mentalhealth.org.uk/a-to-z/d/diet-and-mental-health (accessed March 2019)

- https://www.mentalhealth.org.uk/statistics/mental-health-statistics-stress (accessed March 2019)

- https://www.nhs.uk/live-well/eat-well/the-eatwell-guide/ (accessed June 2019)

- https://www.nhs.uk/live-well/exercise/exercise-health-benefits/ (accessed July 2019)

- https://www.nhs.uk/news/mental-health/fast-food-linked-to-depression/ (accessed April 2019)

- https://www.nutrition.org.uk/healthyliving/healthydiet/healthybalanceddi

References

et.html?1 (accessed April 2019)

- https://www.sciencedirect.com/science/article/pii/S0261561418325408 (accessed September 2019)

- https://www.stress.org.uk/what-is-stress/ (accessed March 2019)

- https://www.takingcharge.csh.umn.edu/why-physical-activity-important (accessed April 2019)

- https://www.theguardian.com/society/2018/sep/26/eating-junk-food-raises-risk-of-depression-says-multi-country-study (accessed June 2019)

- https://www.webmd.com/diet/how-much-water-to-drink#1 (accessed June 2020)

- https://www.who.int/dietphysicalactivity/physical_activity_intensity/en/ (accessed March 2019)

- https://www2.mmu.ac.uk/news-and-events/news/story/?id=9149 (accessed December 2019)

- http://www.health-e-ame.org (accessed May 2020)

- https://www.mentalhealth.org.uk/a-to-z/d/depression (accessed December 2020)

-

Printed in Great Britain
by Amazon